Hist[illegible]
The University of Kansas
School of Medicine-Wichita
1970-2003

by Craig Miner

History of
The University of Kansas
School of Medicine-Wichita
1970-2003

KU SCHOOL OF MEDICINE WICHITA

by Craig Miner

History of The University of Kansas School of Medicine-Wichita 1970-2003
by Craig Miner

Distributed by:
University of Kansas School of Medicine-Wichita Medical Practice Association
1010 N. Kansas
Wichita, Kansas 67214-3199
Phone: (316) 293-2620
Web address: http://wichita.kumc.edu/mpa.html
E-mail: mpa@kumc.edu

Library of Congress Control Number 2005901561

ISBN #0-9762816-0-0

Edited by Regina A. Roths
Cover photo by Brian Atteberry

Photos courtesy of: University of Kansas School of Medicine-Wichita; University of Kansas School of Medicine, History and Philosophy of Medicine Department, University of Kansas Medical Center Archives; University of Kansas, Office of University Relations; and Azim Studios.

Printed in the U.S.A. by Mennonite Press, Inc., Newton, Kansas

Contents

Preface

For some years now, many considered the need to record the history of the University of Kansas School of Medicine-Wichita (KUSM-W). Such a document, it was thought, would not only provide a greater understanding of how and why the school came to be, but also instill a sense of pride in its formation and serve to guide its future direction.

Crafting such a piece, it was realized, would require many hours of research and dozens of interviews with persons involved in the school's formative years.

To take on such a task, the sponsoring organization, the University of Kansas School of Medicine-Wichita Medical Practice Association, approached Craig Miner, Ph.D., distinguished professor of history at Wichita State University, former chair of the Department of History, and author of six publications of local historical prominence. Miner, it was felt, would apply the same rigorous standards of primary and secondary research to this work as with each of his past projects.

The choice was a good one, according to Dr. William Rieke, KUMC's first Executive Vice Chancellor for Health Affairs, who commented upon reading the completed manuscript, "I believe Dr. Miner demonstrates thorough understanding of this complex subject and that his comprehensive research is especially commendable."

Two organizations must also be recognized for their roles in this project, as well as many additional projects over the years. The KUSM-W Dean's Club, a group of supporters contributing to the school's efforts, and the Kansas Health Foundation, a private philanthropy dedicated to improving the health of Kansans, generously provided the financial assistance that made this book possible.

We hope you enjoy reading the result of Miner's efforts, for contained within these pages is a portrait of leadership, a written record of the concerted efforts of local physicians, hospital officials, and administrators from the University of Kansas Medical Center and Wichita State University. Their decisions provided for the school's development in its early years, and continue to be instrumental in its growth over time.

—Garold Minns, M.D.
President
University of Kansas School of Medicine-Wichita
Medical Practice Association

SIGILLUM UNIVERSITATIS KANSIENSIS ©

VIDEBO · VISIONEM · HANC · MAGNAM · QUARE · NON · COMBURATUR · RUBUS

ESTABLISHED 1865

Foreword

Craig Miner's history of the University of Kansas School of Medicine-Wichita (KUSM-W) is a wonderful account of the conception, birth, and growth to adulthood of this important component of the Kansas health care system. The University of Kansas (KU) is very proud of its Wichita School of Medicine and all that has been accomplished in the last thirty years. It is appropriate to commemorate this anniversary with an account of KUSM-W's institutional history.

It is a story that has everything—conflict, drama, bureaucracy, selfless dedication, and competitive behavior. In short, it has all the things that accompany human progress; it details all the fits and starts that attend the beginnings of any success story.

I believe KUSM-W is a noble enterprise, one that Wichita and the state of Kansas should be justifiably proud of creating. It was not easy. There were turf battles, raw politics, and regional jealousies.

Because it was a fundamentally new concept, there were fears that it was too novel. Because it was a different model of medical education, there were questions about its quality. And because it was created in a state that, for the past century, has been hard-strapped for cash, there was an ever-present anxiety over whether the funds to move ahead would be forthcoming.

In the end, the enterprise itself prevailed, as is customary in Kansas, because the dedication of the people involved was stronger than the regional suspicion or the institutional politics.

Today, KUSM-W trains 110 third- and fourth-year medical students with a full-time faculty of fifty-eight and over 900 volunteer faculty from the Wichita community. In addition, 260 medical school graduates serve in thirteen different residencies in Wichita hospitals, all under the sponsorship of KUSM-W.

There was an inexorable logic that led to the founding of KUSM-W and which has continued to the present day. As Robert Hudson, the long-time leader of KU's History of Medicine Department, put it: "Clinical teaching requires a large patient population, and on this Wichita was unchallengeable." Wichita had patients, and KU medical students needed patients if they were to learn their craft. Medical education is highly dependent on clinical teaching. Doctors learn firsthand from other doctors, treating live patients, so that young doctors, when they being practice, can diagnose and treat illnesses first seen in training.

The success of KUSM-W has been shaped by the multitude of opportunities created by the volunteer faculty of the medical practice community of Wichita. Beginning with the hospital-based residency programs that preceded the founding of KUSM-W, Wichita private practice physicians have been the mainstay of medical education in Wichita. The four major hospitals of the late 1960s—Veterans Administration, St. Francis, St. Joseph, and Wesley—worked with the practicing physicians to offer a unique environment for both graduate medical education and undergraduate medical education.

Miner's book is filled with the names of pioneer Wichita physicians who created an "educational culture" in the hospitals where they worked, and this culture greatly facilitated the founding of KUSM-W.

The school really began in 1970 with the creation of a College of Health Related Professions at Wichita State University. Dr. Cramer Reed, a Wichita urologist, became both dean of the school and dean of KUSM-W, the local person in charge of planning for a School of Medicine "branch" in Wichita.

Reed's stewardship of this vision was central to KUSM-W's early success. As Miner says, Dr. Reed "bridged the gaps between WSU, KU, the Wichita medical community, KUMC [the University of Kansas Medical Center], and the state legislators. Reed's personality and aims set the tone and the direction." With accreditation of the Wichita campus in 1974, Reed's dream came true, and he proudly watched the first class receive diplomas in May 1975. Although he left his position as vice chancellor of KUSM-W in 1978, the school was established and the programs were on sound footing. Reed left a solid foundation for his successors and they have built on that foundation.

Deans Richard Walsh, William Reals, Joe Meek, and now Ed Dismuke, have shepherded KUSM-W, with help from strong leaders like Daniel Roberts, George Farha, Anne Walling, Garold Minns, and many others.

Today, any turf battles between KU and WSU have receded into history, and the two institutions consciously look for ways to cooperate. The 110 students each year who receive their third- and fourth-year medical training in Wichita, after early training in basic sciences in Kansas City, realize that they have the best of both worlds. The nearly 300 residents who train in Wichita each year, as part of the Wichita Center for Graduate Medical Education program, have become a major source of doctors for the state of Kansas.

KUSM-W today honors its origins with its dedication to its purpose; relations between the school, the city of Wichita, and KUMC colleagues in Kansas City could not be more positive. Under the careful eye of the medical school accreditation agency, mutually supportive programs have made Wichita a special place for training. The success of KUSM-W speaks for itself, as does all the hard work and dedication that has led to its success.

As Chancellor, I greatly respect the Wichita achievement and the combination of talent and energy that have made it such a vital part of the University of Kansas and the Kansas health care system. We can all take pride in KUSM-W's accomplishments. There is no better way to express that pride than to honor its history.

—Chancellor Robert Hemenway
The University of Kansas

History of
The University of Kansas
School of Medicine-Wichita
1970-2003

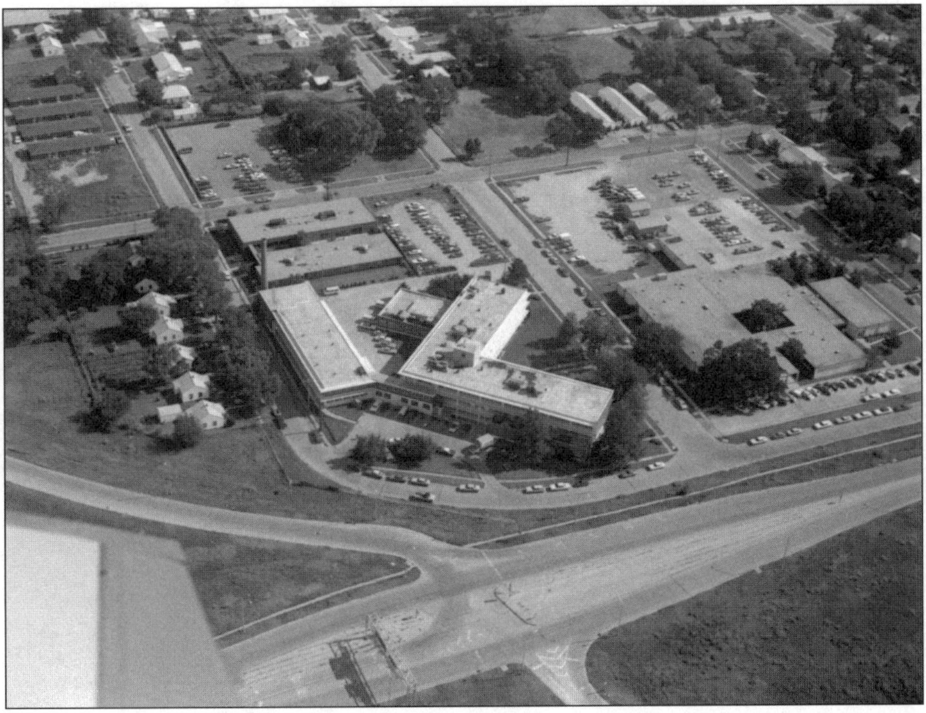

Chapter One

The Case for Wichita

In Kansas, for ever so long, two great centers of state pride have abided—one populous, industrialized, and centrally located; the other only medium-sized, but hoary with state historical tradition, weighted with cultural influence, and able symbolically to survey the intellectual lowlands of the rest of Kansas from the university towers on Mount Oread, which none dared point out was only a hill.

Neither Wichita nor Lawrence was the capital of Kansas. That honor had gone to Topeka, whose Indian name referred to its suitability for growing potatoes. But by the middle of the twentieth century both were clearly the capital of something in the Sunflower State. Wichita had not even been incorporated when the University of Kansas (KU) began developing at Lawrence or when William Quantrill raided the city in 1863, making Lawrence in many ways the martyr city of the "Bleeding Kansas" freedom struggle. Fairmount College at Wichita did not appear until 1895. Its successor institution became Wichita State University (WSU) in 1964 after a bitter struggle in a state legislature filled with University of Kansas alums. KU, however, retained most of the graduate programs, the research presence, the law school, the medical school, and the educational prestige in the state.

But Lawrence had largely missed the boat when it came to the seamy business of moneymaking, a field where Wichita's entrepreneurs excelled. From its time as a rowdy cattle town in the 1870s, Wichita had been criticized for evading some of the state's puritanical standards, including the enforcement of the prohibition amendment, but was given a grudging admiration for its economic drive. Its status as "Air Capital of the World" was firmly established by the late 1920s, when it was manufacturing over 50 percent of the general aviation airplanes in the world. World War II, when $2 billion in federal defense money came to Kansas, mostly to

Wichita, pushed the city's population to over 200,000 and enhanced its wealth. Furthermore, its businesspeople spoke for more than aviation, for they had developed with especial flair railroads, mills, gasoline lamp manufactories, healing salve, fast food franchises, and hospitals. It was a "live" town, as the newspapers once put it, making up in verve what some said it lacked in sophistication.

There could be a rousing "Tale of Two Cities" written about Lawrence and Wichita over more than one hundred years, different as they were, yet linked at the center of the heart and soul of Kansas trying to prosper in a changing world. There is a special case, however, of their being thrown together, not altogether willingly at first, which illustrates especially well both the dynamic of the competition between the two centers of Kansas power as well as the dominant pragmatism of Kansans when it comes to adapting to change. That case is the creation and growth of the University of Kansas School of Medicine-Wichita (KUSM-W) between 1970 and the turn of the twenty-first century.

The 1960s were a time of great change in general, but prominently in medicine. The deep modifications in the health care delivery and finance system brought about by the federal legislation creating Medicare and Medicaid were the most visible aspects of the sea change. But the implications for hospitals and physicians, insurers and patients, and medical schools and their students coming out of the health initiatives of the Great Society program, and out of the societal evolution to which those programs were a response, were to be more profound over time than the most hopeful reformers or fearful traditionalists imagined. They reached and affected everyone, of whatever economic class or political outlook, and in whatever section they lived.[1]

There was a special flux in the field of medical education. The increase in knowledge in the medical field after World War II created a fragmentation of knowledge, an emphasis in residencies on specialties and subspecialties, and a consequent de-emphasis on general practice. Private practice for the first time competed effectively in specialized care with the academic hospitals. Physicians were less likely to be attracted either to an academic career or to general practice in a small town, partly because of the growing gap in income between these callings and specialist private practice. Residencies, which, of course, represented graduate education combined with significant hospital service, burgeoned; biomedical research, with its massive federal funding, became more important; and the emphasis on teaching medical students declined. Reports on medical education as early as 1953 warned that many schools were building "large empires" choosing size over quality in the education of medical students. It was not so much that research did not potentially contribute to good teaching as that, as one historian put it, "student affairs occupied a position of diminishing importance in the institutional value system." At the same time, the curriculum, forced to be aggressively technical, gave little attention to issues such as preventive medicine, occupational medicine, the doctor-patient relationship, and the economic environment in which doctors practiced medicine as a business. Meanwhile, as people began to demand health care as a right, the doctor shortage increased. The Surgeon General's Consultant Group on Medical Education, the so-called "Bane Report," held in 1959 that there would be a nationwide shortfall of nearly 40,000 physicians by 1975.[2]

The decade of the 1960s only intensified both the problems and the study of them. Within a few months in 1966 appeared a spate of significant national reports addressing not only the physician shortage and distribution problem, but also potential solutions. The Willard Report, sponsored by the Ad Hoc Committee on Education for Family Practice at the American Medical Association (AMA), laid the groundwork for a family practice specialty and residencies. The Millis Commission Report addressed the necessary continuum in medical education and the need for better integration of M.D. education and residencies, suggesting the possible elimination of some forms of internships. The Folsom Report, entitled "Health as a Community Affair," helped establish a national "climate of opinion" for the decentralization of medical education.[3]

The distance from Washington, D.C. to Kansas in no way insulated the Sunflower State from the sweep of national trends, as might have been the case at some earlier time. Dr. Gayle Stephens, who was an innovator in the new family practice specialty in Wichita and in establishing one of the nation's first family practice residencies at Wesley Hospital in the late 1960s, commented that the innovations in Wichita in medical education in that era did not represent "reinventing the wheel, just polishing it up locally." The Wichita and Kansas developments, he thought, were part of a "reform movement of many dimensions" in place in medical education from the late 1950s forward.[4]

Kansas had been recognized nationally as a leader in health care and particularly in public health education since the early twentieth century. Dr. Samuel Crumbine, one of the most articulate publicists among physicians anywhere, headed both the Kansas State Board of Health and the University of Kansas School of Medicine in Kansas City, which will hereafter be referred to as KUSM. He had both advanced the health care delivery and medical education system in the state and advertised these to the extent that they were admired and copied elsewhere. His "Swat the Fly" and "Bat the Rat" campaigns, as well as his work against venereal disease in World War I, were internationally known.[5]

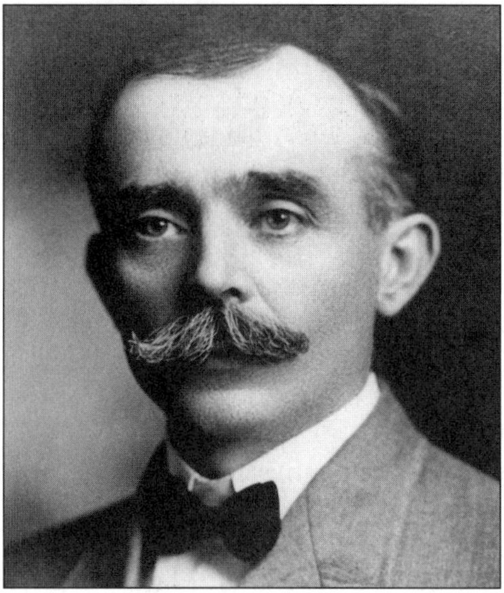

Samuel Crumbine, M.D.

Nor had the state fallen into a medical backwater in the mid-twentieth century. Dr. Ned Burkett of Kingman, for example, became president of the Kansas Academy of General Practice (established 1948) in 1953. He had pushed then, both regionally and in several important national venues, for some of the changes, including board certification for a family practice specialty that came into such prominence in the 1960s.[6] The era of "future shock," however, suddenly required that some long-standing problems in Kansas medicine be faced immediately lest the world move on to the disadvantage of health care there. Looming large among these was the question of the future of medical education in Kansas, a question that was closely related to the quality, focus, distribution, and quantity of physicians practicing there.

The University of Kansas School of Medicine had long been a source of regional pride. Physically located in Kansas City, Kansas, but controlled from the main campus at Lawrence, it began in 1905 as a full-fledged, four-year institution, advancing a two-year course in medicine that had

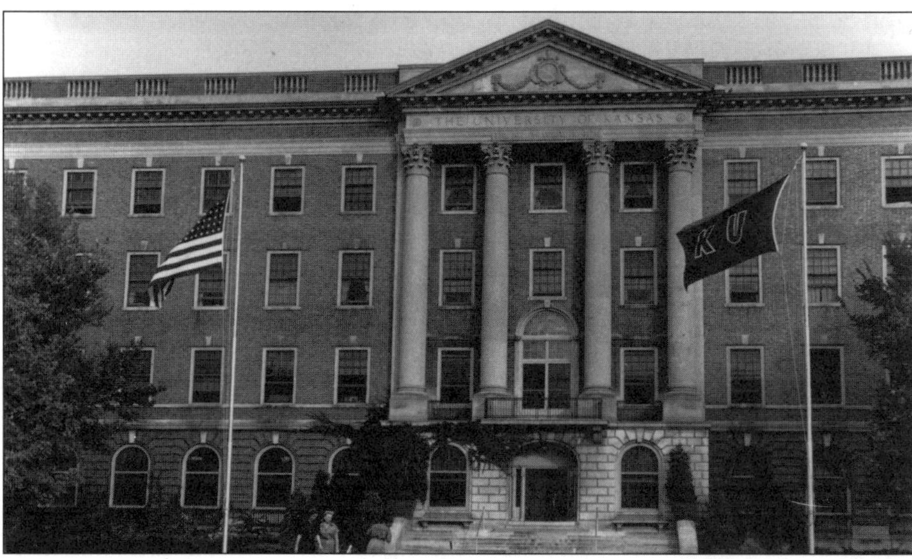

Bell Memorial on the KUSM campus in Kansas City in the 1960s.

existed at the main KU campus since 1880. A small hospital and many ancillary structures arose thanks to substantial contributions by a state legislature that was in the vanguard of the progressive movement in many ways. In 1924, the school moved to a location more elegant than the "Goat Hill" region of its origin. Its new teaching hospital, the Bell Memorial, constructed at a cost of over $235,000, seemed an adequate response to the criticisms that had been directed at the KU School of Medicine in Abraham Flexner's influential 1910 report, *Medical Education in the United States and Canada.*[7]

However, by the mid-1960s, that Kansas City facility, while well respected, was in need of some physical upgrading. Its condition was the result of a period of state political controversy beginning directly upon its completion followed by years of niggardly appropriations from the legislature bottoming in a long dark time through the Great Depression. The state legislature was concerned that rural areas in Kansas, particularly on the high plains in the west, were "underserved" medically. There was also a feeling in Topeka that not enough new physicians were being produced at the KU School of Medicine overall, and that the mix tended to be heavy on specialists who gravitated to urban areas with well-equipped hospitals rather than the "general practitioners," or what had begun to be called the "family practice" specialty, that small towns needed.

One focus was on the training of paraprofessionals in health care at schools of applied health or health-related professions. There was the thought that doctors in the future would increasingly work in specialist groups and clinics, and some of the care delivery heretofore done exclusively by medical doctors would be handled by physicians' assistants and by well-trained nurses. This might be particularly important in addressing the doctor shortage in small towns. A health care assistant might take care of the day-to-day operation of a small-town office, aided by the emerging computer technology that allowed instant communication with urban hospitals and physicians. Then, perhaps, an M.D. could hold consultations twice a week or so, almost like the circuit-riding preachers and judges of an earlier era.

A second thought was that the training of a larger supply of physicians, more oriented toward family practice, could be done less expensively than otherwise by decentralizing medical education. Rather than expanding the university hospital campuses, set as they were on expensive real estate in major cities and loaded as they were with the equipment required for their research agenda, there could be established "branch" campuses in cities remote from the main institution.

These branches could utilize several new techniques. First, they could provide only the last two years of the four-year medical school curriculum

—the "clinical" part. This would avoid reproducing the "basic science" facilities present only in a major university and required for the first two years. Second, and partly because the focus was on clinical rotations, the branch schools could be "community-based." That is to say that, instead of creating a teaching and research hospital exclusively for the university, the branch institution would construct only an administrative center, using the existing community hospitals, with their wide variety of patients, as the setting for the students' experience of such fields as surgery, internal medicine, pediatrics, and obstetrics and gynecology. The faculty at such schools, especially if they were located, as it was expected they would be, in major cities that did not have medical schools, could be drawn from physicians already practicing there who were members of the local medical society. Rather than being full-time academics, many of these doctors might continue their practices and work at the medical school part time. Or, they might even participate in droves, but at a minimal level of commitment of time, as volunteer faculty.

There was much that was controversial about these plans and scenarios and, as of 1970, there was little experience in implementation. However, the Lawrence/Kansas City/Wichita nexus seemed almost the perfect candidate for moving in that direction. The Flexner criticism of the KU operation in 1910 had been that it was a campus divided in two (things were not wholly consolidated in Kansas City until 1962) and that, like so many medical schools then, it depended too much on the old apprenticeship system of observation, and not enough on rigorous academic training. Of course, there were some who believed that any community-based decentralization would be reintroducing sixty years later those same weaknesses with a vengeance.

However, it was a new day and a new set of problems. Wichita had been identified by a Carnegie Foundation study as one of the cities in the United States with the best potential to support a full-scale, four-year medical school.[8] There had been discussion of that possibility in the local medical society off and on since the 1920s.[9]

The prospect of Wichita's developing a competing full medical school on the heels of getting its municipal university accepted into the state system was certainly less attractive to the University of Kansas than a branch of some sort in the metropolis to the southwest. The one history of the KU Medical Center (admittedly primarily a pictorial one) that covered the era of the Wichita connection, made short shrift of the whole matter, but made the threat of a Wichita-controlled competitor seem the whole motive for changes at the KU School of Medicine. After quoting the Kansas City Star's 1958 response to the physician shortage problem that "we need many good doctors, but not one more poorly trained doctor," the history stated that "to head off the possibility of a rival state-supported medical school in Wichita, the Medical Center opened a branch campus in that city in 1971."[10] The story was enough more complicated than that, based as it was on more than intrastate urban rivalries, to justify a deeper historical look at the single question of the evolution of the Wichita campus of the University of Kansas School of Medicine.

The fears of the University of Kansas about Wichita's ambition for a freestanding medical school had some basis early, even though the idea was always a long shot. Wichita did have hospitals to use for the clinical years as well as a substantial university where, with a little expansion, the

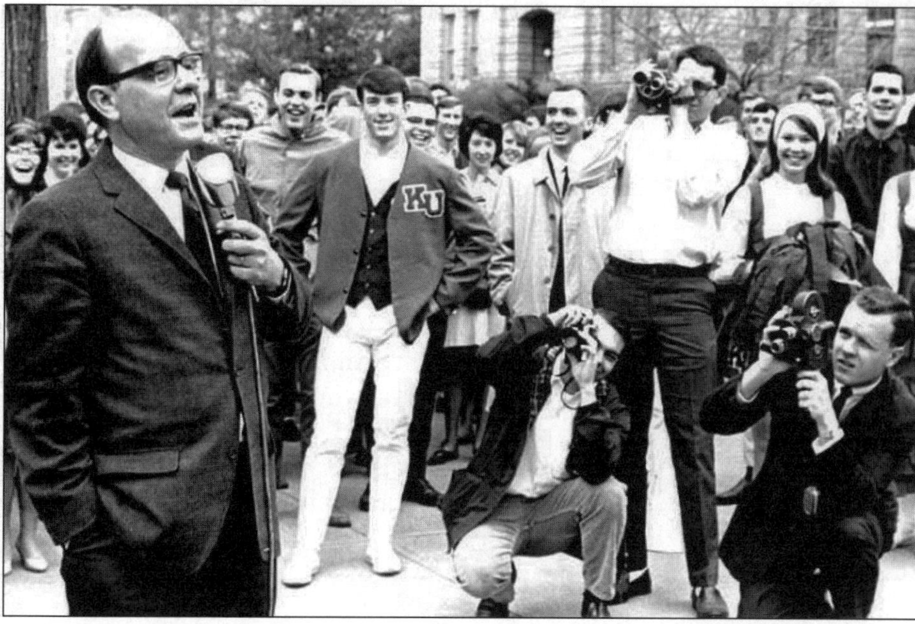

Chancellor Clarke Wescoe with a group on campus.

basic science early years of a medical education could be offered. KU was also frustrated that the Kansas state legislature would consider a "branch" campus on which to center these new initiatives of the 1960s, rather than doing it all in Kansas City. After all, while there had not been the massive modernization on the KU Medical Center (KUMC) campus that was doubtless required, considerable state money was directed there in the 1950s under the leadership of two activist deans, Dr. Franklin Murphy and Dr. Clarke Wescoe. Certainly, there was a recognition of the need for training more physicians and for upgrading the skills of rural general practitioners. The first 100-student class started in Kansas City in 1949. Murphy instituted a program, funded by the Kress Foundation of New York and matched by state funds, to bring general practitioners back to the medical center for one month a year to brush up on the latest medical advances. Senior students from 1950 on were required to spend several weeks as an observer in the office of a rural general practitioner in a community of 2,500 or less. The rural doctors served as preceptors and students accompanied them on their rounds. There were circuit courses as well that took refreshers to the doctors where they practiced. In 1950, the medical center instituted a "geographical full-time" status that allowed faculty members to see patients three afternoons a week in their offices and charged them 7 percent of their income for overhead and another 11 percent for development of their departments. Consequently, from 1947 to 1960, operating income grew from $2,393,000 to $9,725,000. There was substantial revision in the 1950s of a curriculum that had remained largely unchanged since the 1920s, and the revision put more emphasis on clinical and practical work as contrasted with classroom instruction. There was also a response to the criticism that medical education was too narrow and technical. Murphy told a conference in 1948 that a doctor "must be a citizen first, a physician second."[11] Why, some must have wondered, did further change along these lines require a separate campus?

Part of the consideration was cost. A "community-based" campus would require only an administrative center to be built with state funding, not a teaching hospital. And such a facility might be staffed by a combination of part-time and volunteer faculty who, while they would not contribute to overhead through an "in-house" clinical practice, in effect would support themselves by their outside practice and would be relatively inexpensive to the medical center. While not all of these would have research credentials, they were experienced clinicians and, it was imagined, gaining clinical experience would be the focus of a final two years of medical school that might be transferred to Wichita. Also there was the relative lack of "clinical material" at the medical center hospital in Kansas City. The original reason for the location of the School of Medicine in Kansas City in 1905 had been the lack of numbers and variety of patient cases to study in the small town of Lawrence. It was still the case that the specialized university hospital in Kansas City drew from a narrower population than did the private hospitals either in Kansas City, Missouri, or in Wichita. They might receive some patients with "exotic" ailments for which their resident research was helpful, but not as broad a spectrum day by day.

There continued to be informal meetings in Wichita about a possible connection with medical education beyond the hospital-based residencies in a limited number of specialties that already existed. There had been a Wichita Medical College connected with Garfield University in Wichita in the late 1880s, but it failed when the real estate boom crashed in the

1890s, and never issued a diploma.[12] The thought, however, remained that a medical school would be an appropriate accoutrement for such a significant metropolitan region. In fact, *Life* magazine ran a two-page spread in 1950 about the outstanding health facilities in Wichita.[13] In 1952, the Wichita Foundation of Medical Research took a formal survey of its membership concerning the practicality of establishing a medical school in the city as a part of the Municipal University of Wichita. Most of the respondents thought such an idea "premature" though they did not reject the eventual desirability of such an institution. One Wichita physician penciled on the survey form: "Too premature for any hint of insinuation. . . . The medical school needs competition but why warn them before we are ready to deliver?"

Most of the 300-plus members of the Sedgwick County Medical Society felt that an educational component would improve quality of patient care and stimulate their own intellectual development. Perhaps there might be a medical school in Wichita someday, or perhaps a connection with the KU School of Medicine, either temporarily or permanently, would accomplish some of these goals. There was an attempt in the 1950s to promote a Wichitan to become dean of the KUSM at Kansas City, but the movement failed because the selected candidate, Dr. Earl Mills, was not interested in applying.[14] Also there was the feeling that KU was discriminating against Wichita in the relationships the city already had with the medical school. In 1952, for example, the *Bulletin* of the Sedgwick County Medical Society complained that Wichita had 1,185 hospital beds accredited for internships, and had been assigned only three interns from the University of Kansas School of Medicine for 1953. Meanwhile, the KUMC hospital in Kansas City, with 375 beds, had received thirty-eight interns. "This outlandish ratio deserves further investigation." Cities and hospitals needed the interns to improve and lack of them would lesson professional standards. KUMC should see that Kansas communities get their fair share and "to do this satisfactorily the medical school must rid itself of the notion that there is only one place where interns can be adequately trained." At the same time, the *Bulletin* noted, "local people must be alert to their responsibilities." One of those responsibilities might be to create the needed educational component locally on their own.[15]

KU did respond. The acting dean at KUSM wrote the *Bulletin* that only eighteen interns had been assigned to Kansas City, not thirty-eight as reported. Also the dean noted that "using influence" when locating interns was difficult as it was a free choice of location. The implication was that senior medical students would not choose to go to Wichita.[16]

Dr. Stan Friesen, who joined the KU Medical School faculty in 1949, remembers visiting Wichita in the early 1950s with Clarke Wescoe, then Dean of the Medical School and later Chancellor of the University of Kansas. Wescoe brought Friesen because Friesen had grown up near Wichita and had many connections there. These included Dr. Thor Jager, a much-respected Wichita diagnostician of national reputation and head of the Wesley Hospital Laboratory. The topic of their discussions was to investigate the feasibility of a clinical branch for the KU School of Medicine in Wichita.[17] Surely given the stir in Wichita at that time about a medical school and the complaints about discrimination by KU against Wichita, the timing of that visit was not accidental. Presumably, either the visit or the local discussions or both calmed the situation and the medical school question returned to the back burner.

Dr. Lew Purinton, who was Director of Medical Education at Wichita's St. Joseph Hospital, recalls that some years later, but several years before there was any formal start for a Wichita medical school connection, a KU chancellor visited Wichita and talked to a group of fifteen or twenty local people about the possibility of a program for the KU School of Medicine in Wichita. Purinton did not support a four-year medical school in Wichita, nor did he think a connection with WSU was practical. But he did remember the KU people saying they needed more clinical beds to help train medical students, and he remembered positive feedback from Wichita people about that possibility.[18]

That, however, is all the "prehistory" of the thing, locked mostly in oral tradition. In fact, the best history of the matter notes that "the first suggestion that a school of medicine be established in Wichita is 'shrouded in the mists' of Kansas antiquity."[19]

By the late 1960s, however, some things can be documented clearly enough. Appropriately it seems to have begun with a statewide planning exercise. A three-volume consulting report appeared in 1968 entitled "A Plan for the Development of Health Resources, State of Kansas," prepared by Booz, Allen & Hamilton, Inc. for the Kansas Legislative Council. These volumes applied many of the early national studies to the state and were specific about action steps. The authors of the report argued that it was high time for a comprehensive study of the health needs of Kansas since one had not been done since a department of health had been authorized in Kansas in 1889. Its recommendations were wide-ranging, including prominently "the coordination and integration of public and private resources in the development of comprehensive health services, strengthening the board of health, creating regional health organizations for Kansas to replace small county jurisdictions, and increasing state financial support for health."[20] There were many specific suggestions ranging from fluoridation of the water supply to prenatal care for the disadvantaged. Among those were several relevant to health education. These included continued emphasis on health education for the public to determine the feasibility of increasing the class size in the existing medical school, to study the feasibility of establishing a center for health services research, to develop plans to increase the number and quality of graduate medical education programs in the state, to establish additional nursing programs both undergraduate and graduate, to develop educational programs for selected allied health personnel in junior colleges, to determine the feasibility of establishing a school for the allied health professions, and to determine the feasibility of establishing a second medical school.[21]

There was a planning group in Wichita in 1968 that focused on one suggestion that seemed possible for the city in the near future, namely, the creation of a College of Health Related Professions (CRHP) at Wichita State University. This group was essentially the Executive Committee of the Southwest Sector of the Kansas Regional Medical Program (KRMP), itself a response to early Booz, Allen & Hamilton suggestions. Its members were local physicians Alfred Hinshaw, William Reals, Thomas Leuellen, and M.E. Jacobson; Roy House, the administrative head of Wesley Hospital; and John Breazeale, the dean of the graduate school at WSU.[22]

This group produced a document in May of 1968 entitled "Paramedical Education Development (a working document)" authored by Breazeale. The plan noted that many groups in the city and at the university had long been interested in such a move, but that "planning for such programs has proceeded very slowly, primarily because there is no one within the hospitals or the University with both the time and adequate training and background to properly document the need for and plan such programs. There is an urgent need for a qualified person to assume responsibility for these developments." Within WSU there were two plans. The first, proposed by Liberal Arts Dean Kelly Sowards, was to request a budget in fiscal year 1970 from the state legislature for the establishment of a College of Health Related Professions and to hire a dean for it. Breazeale felt this was a flawed strategy, partly because it would involve a direct approach to the Kansas State Board of Regents, perhaps opening Pandora's Box in state politics and second, because WSU had not developed the kind of documentation needed to justify such a program. It was a classic chicken and egg problem. The second idea considered by the working group was to apply for a grant from the KRMP to hire a "regional paramedical education planner," and a secretary for eighteen to twenty-four months, to plan and justify an eventual CHRP. This person should have an M.D. or Ph.D. and would become dean of any college that emerged from this planning. Breazeale's committee therefore suggested this approach to WSU President Emory Lindquist. Breazeale thought the creation of a health-related professions college had much to recommend the university. First, the approach he suggested would not commit a new WSU president to anything beyond the planning stage. Second, it would provide for a two-step approach to the regents while creating "a vehicle for a most desirable kind of community identification with and support of the university in an area other than athletics."[23]

President Lindquist of WSU contacted Chancellor Wescoe with a version of this plan in June. He stated that it had come out of "discussions and interests by the local committee involved in planning." However, he himself was non-committal. "The material has been prepared," he wrote, "at the request of a number of University personnel who feel that it is essential that some kind of coordination be given to a variety of programs on this campus." Those included a proposed nursing program and one in dental hygiene. "There is a feeling that there are federal funds available for support of some of these activities, but that lack of any centrality of direction and planning makes it impossible to secure these funds." Lindquist added, "I feel it is my duty to transmit this matter," though he said, "I do not have enough knowledge at this point to have a valid opinion. . . . I can see some merit in making a study, but it would be my feeling that the study would not be related to any direct implication that it would be implemented because a variety of factors most certainly are involved. This document, as well as many other items from time to time, indicate quite clearly that some vital decisions must be made as to what resources are going to be available for higher education in Kansas as well as the role of this university in the pattern of the future." Lindquist wondered whether "some other organizational pattern" besides a WSU College of Health Related Professions might serve the same ends.[24] In August, Lindquist followed up on this amid internal discussions of the idea in Lawrence and Kansas City.[25]

Wescoe was well aware of the problems addressed both by the Booz, Hamilton report and the Wichita proposal. A year earlier, he had studied a document produced by the University of Vermont College of Medicine concerning the need for physicians in rural areas in that region. Entitled "Eager Communities and Reluctant Doctors," it illustrated that "the current 'crisis in medicine' in the United States has had a long gestation, marked by increasing specialization, proliferation of medical technologies, greater reliance upon hospital facilities and an accelerating 'drift' of physicians from rural to urban areas." The general practitioner was disappearing, and the "old fashioned patient" was also become rare in the age of preventive medicine and wonder drugs. The country doctor had been a "central figure in rural society," but this figure "beloved and overworked, underpaid and idolized," was about gone. The report suggested that this person would be replaced by paraprofessionals—"public health nurses, medical social workers, and variously trained assistants." To accept these would require "increased understanding and attitude changes by the public, not to mention enthusiastic acceptance by the medical profession." Neither would be easy to achieve. Wescoe's reaction to the report was to write, "in many ways it is depressing. On the other hand I think it does give indication that the problems of rural areas will never be solved by giving them more doctors. What we have to do is provide some imaginative program for the delivery of health care based around the regional physician. I would hope that we would be the first to work it out."[26]

The person to whom Chancellor Wescoe addressed these thoughts was Dr. George Wolf, provost and dean at KUSM. He also forwarded Lindquist's June 1968 letter about the WSU plan for health-related professions. "There is no hurry about it," he said in his cover letter, "but I thought you should be informed and that we should have a response ready."[27]

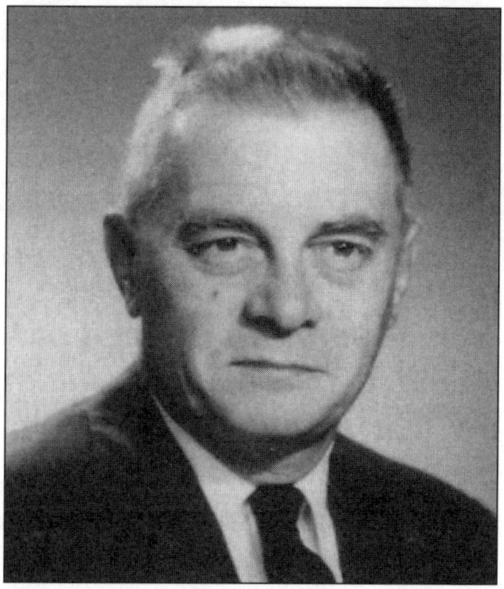

George Wolf, M.D., KUSM Provost and Dean

One unusual event, the explanation for which goes deeper than any documentation, was that Wolf and Wescoe right away offered Lindquist, who was stepping down as president of WSU, a position at the University of Kansas School of Medicine. The offer was by telephone, so no details remain in the archives. Lindquist in a handwritten reply (he had no longer a secretary or IBM Selectric) said he wanted to return to classroom teaching where he might be able to introduce students to the "tradition of civility."[28] What suitability Lindquist, whose academic background was history, might have had for KUSM can only be guessed. Similarly speculative would be what political advantage, if any, such a shift might have been expected to provide. One possibility is that there was a thought of a closer connection between the School of Medicine and Wichita State University and that having a former president of WSU, who had exercised a masterful diplomacy with the state legislature in the wake of the contentious entry of that university into the state system, might be helpful. Lindquist was the quintessential moderate, the truly "civil" man who had a broad view of the complexity of things and tended not to act as a narrow partisan. That kind of prestige and connection in the KU camp at the beginning of a time of flux could help. Something big was going to happen to health care in Kansas, and Wichita, with its large population, wide range of physicians, and strong hospitals, was bound to be in the game.

Chapter Two

From Root to Branch

From these tentative plans arose in a very short period of time, not only a College of Health Related Professions at Wichita State University, but a much expanded group of residencies in Wichita hospitals and a "branch" of KUSM located on the campus of Wichita State and designed to educate a growing class of medical students in their final two clinical years. Surely this was both promising and frustrating to university officials in Lawrence and Kansas City. Dr. Robert Hudson commented: "The Wichita proposal resurrected some of the same arguments heard when the main university went to Lawrence and the Medical School to Kansas City." Here, just when the dream of unifying the KU Medical School all in one place seemed a possibility there came another geographical split. And just when it seemed that the dream of centralized control and a standard curriculum was near, came decentralization and a sort of bifurcated mission. While Hudson contended that the Wichita discussion was never "as, shall we say, colorful" as those over the previous split, it had its drama. But at least there was a strong reason for the Wichita branch and it was logistical. "Clinical teaching requires a large patient population, and on this Wichita was unchallengeable. This is not to say the move was hailed uniformly in Kansas City, or the rest of the state, for that matter. But all considered, the Wichita move was accomplished with a relative lack of stridor."[29] Yes, perhaps, "all considered."

It all started with the utmost politeness and at the most modest conceivable level. Wolf told Wescoe in the summer of 1968 that he thought it was a good idea for Wichita University (KU administrators for a time continued to call Wichita State by its former name as a municipal institution) to develop an allied health program in conjunction with the University of Kansas. Matters would be "complicated" by a change of presidents in Wichita, but Wolf had met the new president, Clark Ahlberg, and knew that Ahlberg had both Washington experience and a background in the financing of medical education. It would be well to meet with the new man. "It may perhaps be a little rough on him to hit him with this soon after his arrival because of the noises made by K-State [Kansas State University, which was proposing a nursing program at the time], our situation and the obvious good position of the University of Wichita as far as clinical facilities are concerned." However, there was promise in the plan, and the two universities might well approach the Kansas Board of Regents together and let that body look at the idea "from the standpoint of the entire university system."[30] In the fall of 1968, Wolf forwarded to Wescoe some germane sections of the Booz, Hamilton recommendations, although he noted that it was "a three volume opus and pretty hard to summarize."[31]

The key combination of events that moved things out of the planning stage seems to have been a series of meetings between two "Clarks"—Clarke Wescoe, who became Chancellor of the University of Kansas in 1960 and Clark Ahlberg, who became president of Wichita State University in 1968.[32] They both presided over tumultuous times for their universities and others and had much on their minds other than medical education. However, both men had a background and interest in medical education. Wescoe, as mentioned, had been Dean of the KU School of Medicine. Ahlberg had been Vice President for Research at Syracuse University, which had an affiliated College of Medicine, and he was a member, too, of the National Institutes of Health's governing council. In both capacities he became well acquainted with medical schools and their funding.[33]

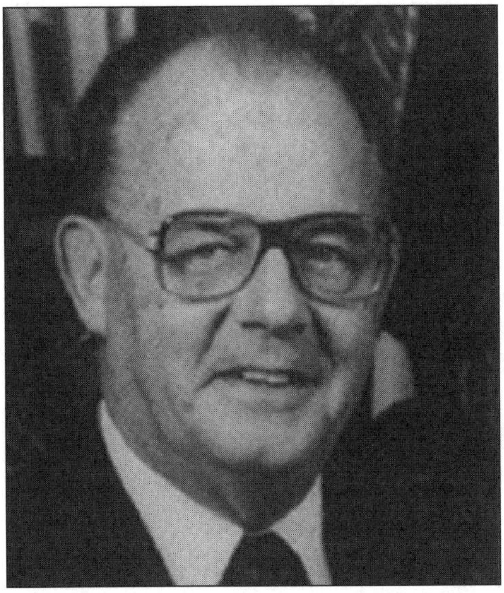

Clark Ahlberg, President, Wichita State University

Ahlberg was the immediate initiator of the talks with Wescoe and Wolf.[34] The WSU president was interested in a "joint venture" with KU. This would serve to stabilize the position of WSU in the state system, which was described at that time by an accrediting agency as "somewhat cloudy."[35] When WSU was the University of Wichita, a municipal institution established in 1926, it had developed a baccalaureate program in nursing and had recently added a dental hygiene program to that. Ahlberg felt this was a basis for expansion in Wichita, and that it was an appropriate start since the move was in the area of training in the health-related professions rather than the more jealously guarded and expensive training of medical doctors. He saw the medical school connection as a chance to define the words "urban-related" in the WSU mission statement and thought that a venture with KU Medical Center was, as John Breazeale, now Vice President for Academic Affairs, put it, "a major and appropriate chance for expansion of Wichita State University."[36]

The *Wichita Eagle* thought so also. It reported favorably in April 1969 on a visit to Wichita by Dr. Darrell J. Mase of the University of Florida. Dr. Mase, a native of Delphos, Kansas, established the first university health department in the nation in 1958. While in town to address the Kansas Psychological Association convention at the Lassen Motor Hotel, he met with Dr. Ahlberg, as he had met with WSU President Lindquist on previous visits. Martin Palmer, who founded the Institute of Logopedics at the University of Wichita in the 1930s had, Mase said, a "concept for taking services to the people." He was criticized for it at the time, but it seemed germane in the 1960s, and in fact was the pattern in the U.S. for health care. Kansas had twenty regional speech centers staffed by personnel trained at Wichita, and Mase thought that could well be a model for serving rural communities in the future. There would have to be paraprofessionals in many roles. "If medical professions are to grow," Mase stated to the local reporter, "doctors, dentists, and others must be willing to give up some of their often jealously guarded duties." Dental hygienists could clean teeth as well as dentists, and the professions were "top heavy with people with advanced degrees, holding on to this as if nobody else could do it, nobody else dared." Colleges were training too many psychologists for academia and research positions and not enough for hospitals, schools, and clinics. Any applied health school must "fit the personality of the university" in which it was housed, Mase thought, but WSU seemed to him to have the ideal sort of personality for this type of school.[37]

Ahlberg, Wescoe, and Wolf talked in 1969 about a cooperative endeavor in Wichita.[38] Wescoe and Ahlberg, according to Ahlberg's friend and administrative associate Dr. George Platt, hit it off well and developed a "superb relationship." The Kansas Board of Regents at that time was much interested in such cooperative relationships, no doubt recognizing that the state had, if anything, too many universities for it to fund adequately. For a time, there had been thought of WSU itself being a branch of KU, with KU professors commuting to Wichita on the

Kansas Turnpike. In the late 1960s, WSU had several joint doctoral programs with KU. These worked smoothly and provided a background for a potential medical relationship.[39]

Out of these discussions grew a planning document entitled "A Proposed College of Health Related Professions, Wichita State University, Feasibility Study." This emerged in the summer of 1969 and the author was Dr. Jack Walker, who was Associate Professor of Community Health and Preventive Medicine and associate dean at KUSM. The discussions of a year earlier had made it clear "that it would be reasonable to pursue a cooperative endeavor." This was true for several reasons. First, there was a severe shortage nationally in all health fields and especially in Kansas. Kansas medical education was limited at the baccalaureate and post-baccalaureate levels for health-related professions and at the internship and residency levels for physicians. Second, there was great potential in Wichita and at Wichita State for a health-related professions college. A "vast array" of clinical health facilities existed in the city and the university had growing enrollments and departments of biology, chemistry, physics, math, and sociology capable of providing "the academic background for the development of education programs in the health-related fields." Third, the Wichita metropolitan area contained 25 percent of the population of Kansas. Fourth, Wichita was far enough from Kansas City to avoid overlap, given the start that already existed there. For these reasons Walker concluded that "it seemed logical and beneficial for Wichita University and the University of Kansas Medical Center to pursue this study of a cooperative endeavor in the best interest of the state of Kansas."[40]

Indeed the training of paraprofessionals in the health field seemed a growing trend. From an origin when the St. Louis University School of Nursing branched out in 1929, the field had grown. The University of Pennsylvania School of Allied Medical Professions began in 1950. The University of Florida College of Health Related Professions came along in 1957, and Indiana University's school in 1958. By 1966, there were thirty such colleges within universities, and it was estimated there would be sixty by the end of 1969.[41]

The need was there. In 1900, there had been one supporting person for each practicing physician. In 1969, the ratio was thirteen-to-one and it was expected to be twenty-to-one by 1975. Although allied health students had historically been trained in hospitals, students and faculty in that field "find themselves in uncomfortable administrative and academic positions in the traditional college or university." Allied health was not a good fit for colleges of liberal arts, and there was no other "reasonable academic" home in the academy as usually then constituted.

"At no time," the feasibility study noted, "have the disparities between the expectations and need for health services and the capacity to supply these services been more obvious." Hospitals would need much more staff and the delivery of health services in rural areas of Kansas was, according to the report, "an increasingly acute problem." The rural population was declining in size but "expect and deserve access to first rate medical and health services. The dilemma over what to do about this situation is taxing the minds of concerned individuals." Attracting more doctors to the state and training more doctors in the state was part of the solution, but training paraprofessionals was just as important.[42]

The existing WSU program consisted of bachelor of science degrees in nursing, medical technology, and logopedics and an associate degree in dental hygiene. The feasibility study proposed adding immediately bachelor of science degrees in physical therapy, occupational therapy, and dietetics and nutrition, and a master's degree in medical technology. In the longer term it would be desirable to have degrees for medical librarians and medical security and perhaps even a college of dentistry.[43]

What about a complete freestanding medical school? The question of

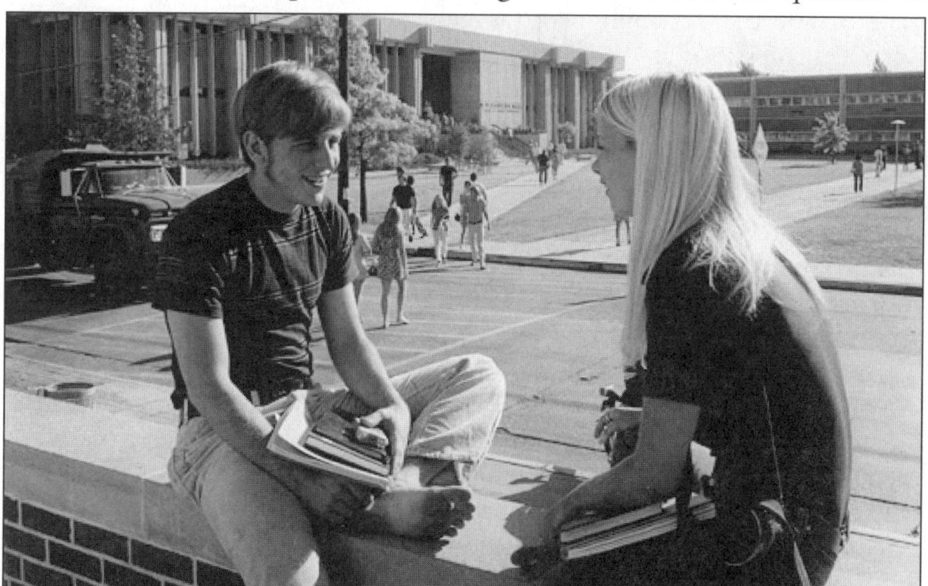

WSU campus in the 1960s.

a medical school located at Wichita State, the report noted "arose many times."[44] The Booz, Hamilton report had recommended studying the "desirability and feasibility" of increasing the class size of the existing medical school, of developing additional internships and residency training programs in cooperation with Kansas hospitals, and of establishing a second medical school.[45] However, the feasibility study came out strongly against a second medical school at WSU or anywhere. KUSM could accommodate classes of 125 at the existing Kansas City campus, and until the academic year 1968–69 the number of qualified applicants from Kansas had always been fewer than that. The recent surge in Kansas applicants, the study claimed, was largely due to selective service deferment policies in the Vietnam War and was not likely to continue. There was indeed a doctor shortage in rural Kansas, but the author of the feasibility study thought there was no reason to believe that the creation of a medical school in southcentral Kansas would make much of a difference in the career choices of doctors. Besides, the cost of a second medical school would be "enormous" and "unrealistic" in the current fiscal climate. Even if the funding were to fall into place, faculty procurement would be a problem. The study concluded, "realistic consideration of the above factors seriously mitigates against the establishment of a second medical school in Kansas at this time." That could change in the future, but for the present, WSU, KU, and KUMC all concurred in these conclusions.[46]

Instead, the feasibility study recommended a College of Health Related Professions at WSU, jointly administered by WSU and KU. The dean of the Wichita college would also be an associate dean for the KU School of Medicine. "This arrangement would be unique and valuable to both institutions and would be in the best interest of promoting educational opportunities and programs in the health fields for the citizens of Kansas." The suggestion was to request $73,642 in fiscal year 1971 for this program, and to begin right away "to bring present programs into coordination with each other." There was a projection that the budget might be nearly $200,000 by 1975.[47]

A second focus should be on expanding residency programs in Wichita. This was especially desirable in that the research indicated a greater correlation between the geographical area where doctors took their residencies and where they decided to practice than there was between the medical school they attended and the locus of their eventual career. Again KU and WSU could cooperate in supporting and expanding these programs, perhaps with the eventual result that the universities would take more of a role in administering these, satisfying the accrediting agencies in contrast to the hospital-based residencies that were thought not to be the trend of the future. Wichita had four major hospitals—the Veterans Administration, St. Francis, St. Joseph, and Wesley. In 1969, these had American Medical Association-approved residencies in internal medicine, surgery, anesthesiology, radiology, pathology, family medicine, obstetrics and gynecology, orthopedic surgery, and urology.[48]

The family medicine residency, housed at Wesley, was an especially important element of Wichita's medical education resources. It had begun in 1967, only a year after the Willard report, sponsored by the Council on Medical Education of the American Medical Association, had suggested the desirability of such residencies. At first, it operated under Wesley's general practice residency until the American Board of Family Practice was approved early in 1969. Organized by Dr. Gayle Stephens, and operated initially out of a small house on Pine Street, it was one of the first such residencies in the nation.[49] Given that training of more family practice physicians was thought by all the reports and studies to be particularly important to address the general doctor shortage and the particular rural doctor shortage in Kansas, the existence of that residency in Wichita was a strong reason for KUMC/WSU/hospital cooperation there in the interest of the entire state.

Stephens himself, however, was suspicious of the motives of the University of Kansas, both at the early stage of enhancing residencies and creating CHRP, and at the later step of establishing a WSU branch of KUSM. He was not untypical in such thinking of many other Wichita physicians and laypeople.

The University of Kansas, Stephens thought, had more of an interest in family practice than many medical schools. Some significant part of the faculty there looked down on it as less heavyweight academically than other specialties, and KUSM had not been moving fast enough in the direction of training more family practice specialists to please the state legislature. "I thought I had a leg up on what primary care meant," Stephens said, "and that was part of the rhetoric for establishing the new school." At one point, a bit later than these initial discussions, there was an appropriation passed by the legislature earmarked for family practice education and outside the KUMC budget. Although it was a nominal amount, it illustrated an intention that was offensive to KU. Stephens's opinion was that KU "was an opportunist in this development. They had usurped an impulse that had grown in Wichita and acted preemptively." Dr. James Donnell, for example, who was on the Wichita City Commission, and who took a great interest in promoting a full-fledged medical school in Wichita "did not have much love for KU," and doubtless the KU administration knew it. Donnell and Stephens thought that the KU people, although, in Stephens's opinion, they had not much enthusiasm for family practice or paraprofessional training, would protect their back by usurping what was percolating in Wichita "and bend it to their own desires."[50] Despite these suspicions in Wichita and parallel counter-suspicions in Lawrence and Kansas City, in 1969 and 1970 implementation of the recommendations of Walker's study did go forward.

Other hospital residencies, where there had already been cooperation in Wichita with the University of Kansas, became the focus of the early development of the new Wichita branch. For example, training in internal medicine had become more standardized and, by the mid-1960s, St. Francis and Wesley developed three-year internal medicine residencies to replace their former one-year programs. The VA Hospital was a Deans' Committee Hospital, which meant the KUSM-W Department of Internal Medicine could oversee the quality of the program. Dr. Ernest Crow of Wichita, who was to become the first chair of the Department of Internal Medicine at the University of Kansas School of Medicine-Wichita, recognized that accreditation for residencies depended increasingly on a university affiliation, and that it would be wise for the other hospitals to join with the VA in seeking such an academic connection. In about 1965, the hospitals started a combined residency with a six-month rotation at KUMC. In October 1969, just as the discussions between WSU, KU, and KUMC were leading to plans for broad cooperation, there was an agreement that specifically defined the relationship with KUMC in regard to the Wichita hospital internal medicine residencies. The Department of Internal Medicine at KUSM in Kansas City agreed to "direct medical residents to the Wichita program," the rotations to Kansas City for Wichita medical residents would continue, and the visiting KUSM faculty program would continue and be enhanced. Dr. Carter Goodpasture, former Director of Medical Education at Wesley, became Director of the Wichita Combined Internal Medicine Residency.[51]

According to Dr. Crow, "Wichita was, in a sense, unique" in its readiness for expanded medical education. Its pioneer physicians—the likes of Drs. Andrew Fabrique, Thor Jager, Earl Mills—were all interested in education and installed an educational culture at the hospitals where they dominated the institutional culture. So there was both a culture and a tradition in Wichita ripe for medical education. There was a desire, as Crow put it, "to in some way get Kansas City to recognize Wichita as a medical community."[52] The hospitals were cooperative, as they liked the idea of the prestige of a medical school connection and of expanding their residency programs. It was a harbinger of future directions.

The next step was the creation of the College of Health Related Professions at Wichita State University. In February 1970, Ahlberg appointed Dr. D. Cramer Reed, a Wichita urologist, as dean of the new CHRP.[53] In April, he became also an associate dean at KUSM.[54]

The parameters of the relationship had been worked out earlier, in December 1969. Ahlberg confirmed with Dr. George Wolf at KU the nature of Reed's responsibilities in order to "avoid misunderstanding." Ahlberg described the positions "as one involving acting for you [Wolf] in this community to represent the University of Kansas Medical Center." Reed would develop cooperative education with the hospitals in Wichita with respect to resident and intern programs. He would assist Wolf and the KU academic departments in the development of "any undergraduate medical relationship involving the hospitals in Wichita." In the area of health-related professions, Reed would be responsible to the president of WSU. "He would, however, be expected to cooperate with the medical center in the development of such programs, particularly in those areas where the medical center is currently operating such programs." It was a dual appointment, in short, "with important status in both institutions but with separate responsibilities to each." He was to be compensated initially for the first twelve months by WSU with the expectation that KUMC would reimburse WSU for one-third of Reed's salary or more depending on what his actual division of labor was.[55]

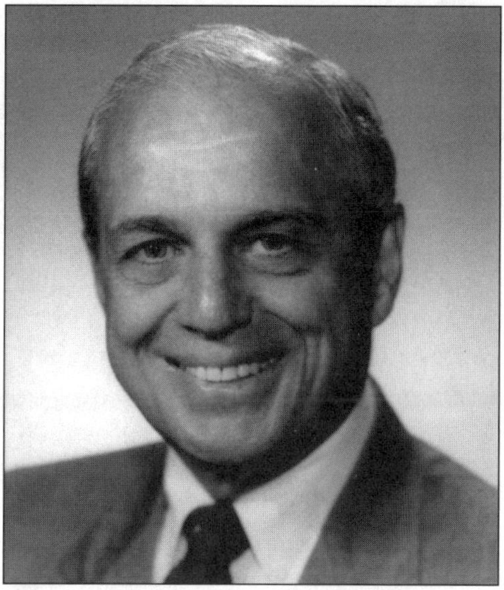

D. Cramer Reed, M.D., became KUSM-W's first dean.

Initial annual funding for CHRP was a modest $70,000.[56] All involved understood, however, that it could be the beginning of something very large. CHRP created cultural changes within the university, in the relationship between WSU and the community of Wichita, and in the relationship between Wichita State University and the University of Kansas.

Within the university, CHRP and other "urban mission" programs, like the Administration of Justice program shortly created with federal grants, diminished the dominance of the College of Liberal Arts and complicated faculty governance by creating an expanded faculty that was less homogeneous in its views and interests. About 80 percent of the students in CHRP by the mid-1970s were women, and there was a higher percentage of women on its faculty as well, leading to women for the first time taking the leadership positions in the faculty senate. But Ahlberg convinced the Department of History, which for a time was in "sackcloth and ashes" over the change, that there were legitimate academic pursuits other than the traditional humanities, and that applied training to meet public needs could and should be a legitimate part of a real university.[57]

WSU always had close ties to its community, but certainly the creation of CHRP and the bringing of Reed, an M.D., not a Ph.D., to administer a new college, created a relationship with physicians that was different. Fred Sudermann, who was on the WSU administrative team at the time, remembered that Ahlberg felt that Reed could pull the health community together and create benefits for the university far beyond simply the support and growth of CHRP. Before, Sudermann said, the only time WSU administrators talked to doctors was "when they wanted money for the athletic department."[58] Physicians were intellectuals with a pragmatic bent, and there was great interest among Wichita physicians in both research and medical education. While they had created research foundations, the presence of a medical school was much missed by the more modern specialists who had trained in major medical centers. Some perceived the health professions initiative as an entering wedge, but many others saw it as a boon in itself.[59]

There were several levels of discomfort for KU in the CHRP expansion and other WSU initiatives. Although Reed was appointed associate dean at KUSM at the same time that he became dean of the College of Health Related Professions at WSU, CHRP was primarily a WSU program, by reason of geography and dominant administrative responsibility.[60] Ahlberg was clearly interested in the growth of the university beyond the strict "urban mission" in Wichita and Sedgwick County to which it seemed confined by its Board of Regents mission statement. "Wichita was always flexing its muscle," remembered Dr. Joseph Meek, who was at KUMC at the time, "and acting bigger than it was entitled to act."[61]

And Ahlberg had both the personal capability and local support to create successful initiatives in that direction. It was a "quiet goal" of his, Ahlberg said in recalling those times, never to abandon the idea that WSU was what its former history had made it, a service institution for Wichita, but also "to do everything possible to broaden our base in the state and create an institution with a base far broader than Sedgwick County." He thought CHRP was a natural for this. He knew all about the aspects for getting funding for such a health program and there was a great need for people to work in fifty-bed hospitals in western Kansas. Reed was well respected around the state as well as in Wichita and could and would negotiate at the highest level with the true power brokers in the legislature and elsewhere. He was also a zealot, but a soft-spoken and diplomatic zealot for the cause that Ahlberg thought was needed to break inertia at home and log jams abroad.

Certainly the other state universities would oppose an invasion of what they considered their turf. Ahlberg noted, however, that people in

Wichita were a little bitter about the opposition of these universities to their entry into the state system, and that the "saddle sores" acquired in that fight made the community supportive of the idea of taking as much advantage as possible of the opportunity of finally being a state university. Perhaps there were some niches, Ahlberg thought, like CHRP and Administration of Justice, that could be developed with federal money and which, as he put it, "were below the dignity of the University of Kansas."[62]

A WSU self-study in 1976 was to state that it was one of an emerging class of "comprehensive regional universities . . . whose vitality attests to their ability to respond, rapidly and flexibly, to new and uncertain situations."[63] Such vitality and flexibility was not necessarily in the interest of KU, especially when the supposed "undignified" programs evolved into direct threats to prime academic territory. There had been all too much recent history in the nation of urban "branches" becoming the monsters that ate the main campus. The Milwaukee campus of the University of Wisconsin, for instance, grew bigger than the Madison campus in Wisconsin and developed a full line of graduate programs. It could happen in Kansas.

Still, people at KUMC and at Lawrence were certainly attuned to the potential of a community-based school and to the desirability of increasing the class. Dr. Charles Brackett, who headed KUMC for a little over a year in 1970–71 following Wolf, recalled later the enthusiasm for the concept. Students, he said, "got to see medicine as it really is, not in the artificial atmosphere of the medical center." There was a volume of clinical material in Wichita, and there was a chance to observe doctors making a living somewhat as a student might in some future practice in a Kansas town.[64]

KUMC, far from ignoring the new needs as beneath its interest, had done considerable planning to try to keep as much of the expansion as possible in Kansas City. It had a way to go. In 1970, the medical center had 535 beds with a budget of $39 million. Much of the clinical facility was out of date and there were only six intensive care beds in the institution. There was an administrative staff of only sixteen for the entire hospital and medical school operation. Dr. George Wolf, recognizing that something would have to be done, had authorized a preliminary study for expansion in Kansas City in 1968, and the report completed by Lester Gorsline Associates suggested accommodating 150 medical students by 1975. Wolf had also been seeking federal funding to increase the size of the class, to increase minority recruiting, and to develop clinical affiliations at Wichita, Topeka, and elsewhere in Kansas City. In addition, there was a thought of reducing the four-year curriculum to a three-year course of study. However, the golden age of federal funding in the Great Society period was coming to an end, and therefore the leadership at KUMC saw special urgency in appealing to the Kansas Board of Regents and the legislature. Further architectural studies were done, and KUMC created, under the supervision of Dr. Robert Manning, a three-volume study called "Education for Health Care in Kansas" that outlined what the health care system in the state might look like in 1980.

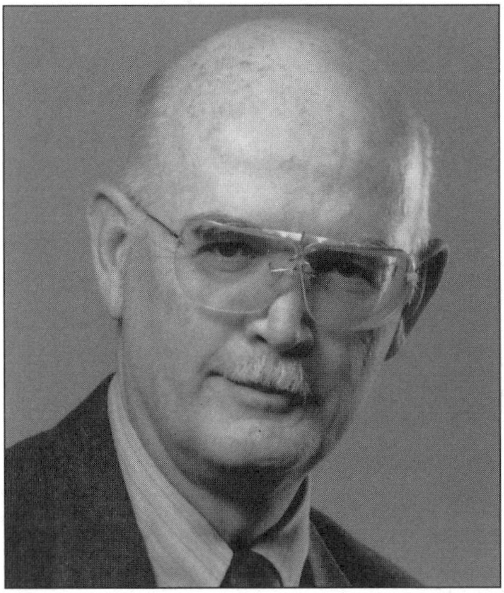

Robert Manning, M.D.

The report recommended support of allied health programs, and suggested that clinical training of 40 percent of KUSM medical students might take place in affiliated programs at Wichita and Topeka covering only the last two, clinical years of their education. It also suggested the construction of a new 450,000 square foot teaching hospital in Kansas City that would include new basic science facilities and 770 beds at a cost of over $60 million. KUMC also moved to develop a program in family practice and, in April 1971, it hired Dr. Jack Walker as the first chairman of the Department of Family Practice.[65]

Wichita was moving also, both to plan the proposed coordination and to absorb as big a piece of the responsibility as it could. Reed had many concerns about the relationship. He made some handwritten notes about 1970, wondering, at least to himself, whether the KUSM faculty was "sufficiently committed to affiliate to make it go—KUMC must lead the way—Wichita is leery and questions sincerity. . . . Some are saying—if eventually, why not now in Wichita." Was KU sensitive to the needs of the western part of the state? "I am concerned over competitive actions of hospitals—could ruin show by each insisting on 'its' own program (hope MSSC [Medical Society of Sedgwick County] response can be positive and recommend community cohesiveness)." The whole thing seemed tenuous. "In view of KUMC faculty reaction and no assurance of funding of expansion project—I get 'nervous' about talking up affiliate. Can only talk of intangibles now—*if* I promote the deal and it falls thru—effectiveness with CHRP may be jeopardized." Meanwhile more local businessmen (Reed mentioned Martin Umansky of KAKE-TV and

Willard Garvey of Garvey Industries) were wondering out loud why Wichita should not have an independent medical school.[66]

Reed wrote Brackett in May 1970 that prior to Wolf's departure in April as provost and dean of the medical school, he, Reed, had been visiting KUMC weekly, making appointments with department heads and attending administrative meetings. He hoped to continue this under Brackett's bridge administration in the interest of "our combined causes." He was interested, he said, in enhancing the relationship between Brackett's office and the CHRP "and want to do whatever is appropriate to do so."[67] Reed contacted Associate Dean Walker about meeting in Kansas City concerning residency requirements.

This helpfulness, as well as the complications that arose as Wichita hospitals joined in the affiliation between the two universities, were viewed with some trepidation in Kansas City. Walker complained to Reed after a recent meeting with Homer Holt, who was requesting residencies at Wichita's St. Francis Hospital for general surgery, internal medicine, and obstetrics and gynecology. Holt and his group, Walker said, "had immediately gone back to Wichita and attempted to find areas in which they could expand their programs. At first glance, one would be inclined to believe that this was unilateral searching for ways and means to obtain part of the funding. This may not be true. I think what we'll have to do is ask these people to very carefully outline for us the justification for such requests including considerable background information on each residency program. . . . I can predict now, that it's going to be a long summer and fall attempting to work out the details with these affiliated programs and attempting to please everyone."[68]

Reed admitted that the residencies were "a very sensitive area in this community," and that Holt appeared "to have made some rather dramatic, and I hope not irresponsible, commitments concerning program implementation at St. Francis Hospital. My problem is that I cannot really find out exactly what he has told these people, and continue to get various rumors which does not make for 'great peace.'"[69] Holt had assured Reed that St. Francis "desires and is eager for close specific affiliation with KUMC," and hoped that Kansas City would assign residents to obstetrics and gynecology and pediatrics, so that those programs could be implemented at his hospital in 1971, perhaps as a combined residency. "The administration of St. Francis Hospital has demonstrated sincere interest and cooperation in attempting to develop and improve medical education in Wichita."[70] Dr. Lew Purinton, who had been director of medical education at St. Joseph Hospital since 1958, was concerned, meanwhile, that most of the residency planning revolved around Wesley and St. Francis Hospital, and that his hospital's active residencies in pathology and family practice might be compromised. He wanted to meet with Reed and the medical education directors at the other hospitals.[71] Purinton was facing a divided staff at his institution in regard to the affiliation with KUMC. Dr. William Reals, head of the pathology residency program, was much in favor of the university association as was the central administration at St. Joseph, but the program directors of the family practice residency were less enthused. They felt the residency would ultimately be entirely controlled by the university, and preferred that it remain independent and hospital-based.[72] Reed wrote Dr. Lester Garfinkel, director of medical education at Wesley Hospital, in the fall of 1970, asking him for information to substantiate the need for financial support to increase KUMC's capacity "and to further implement the relationship of the Wichita training hospitals as major teaching affiliates of the medical center." He recognized, he said, that predicting to 1980 could involve at best "gross approximations," but they needed to try. Reed asked if Garfinkel would really want an association with KUMC. He doubted whether the legislature would approve a five-year package, data or no data, and noted that the whole thing "could be submarined at any point."[73] Dr. Daniel Roberts at Wesley provided some statistical information to the chair of obstetrics and gynecology at KUMC, adding, "since I'm sure you are well aware of the multiple problems that are developing in terms of the affiliations and/or associations of the Wichita hospitals with KU, I will not need to explain the slow movement that seems to be taking place in the formation of our relationship."[74] The question for Reed was how all the interests were to be balanced and where the central initiative lay. He began making himself handwritten lists of things to ask on his next visit to Kansas City.

The potential significance of Wichita in a future expansion program was further underscored when Dr. Charles Brackett, the acting Vice Chancellor for Medical Affairs at the University of Kansas Medical Center, and Dr. Reed from Wichita State University, appeared together before the Kansas Board of Regents in November 1970. The topic was a five-year plan to start meeting the physician shortage in Kansas. The alternatives presented were expansion of KUMC at a cost estimated at over $50 million, the creation of a new medical school at Wichita State University, or possibly both.[75]

Brackett preferred option one, but said that "if the KU Medical Center is not able to accommodate expansion by 1975 that consideration be given to creation of a second medical school in Wichita." Meanwhile he supported the idea of increasing the number of interns and residents in Wichita hospitals and recommended that Wichita State be permitted to offer associate of arts, two-year degrees in certain medical areas. The

Regents had a special meeting in Wichita and looked over documents indicating that there was an immediate need for over 500 active practicing physicians in Kansas and that the shortfall would reach 1,386 by 1980.[76] About 30 percent of Kansas physicians had reached the last decade of their expected professional life, and it was thought that, by 1980, twenty-two counties would have to replace half or more of their physicians.[77]

Should there be a need for a second medical school in Wichita, Dr. Brackett estimated it would cost $25 million and could handle seventy students. Both Brackett and the Regents were aware of a report by the Carnegie Commission on Higher Education, just issued that October, that listed Wichita among the top urban possibilities as reasonable sites for new medical schools.[78] Brackett testified that "responsibility for health education must be spread through the state," whether or not that spreading involved a full-fledged second medical school in Wichita.[79]

In February 1971, Dr. Reed appeared before the Board of Directors of the Medical Society of Sedgwick County (MSSC). What shape the future of medical education in Kansas would take, he emphasized, would depend to some extent on the attitude of the Society. He pointed out that the creation of a second medical school in Wichita was only one "of several alternative possibilities," but it was a definite possibility. The University of Kansas was putting a $54 million expansion package before the 1971 legislature, and a bill would "likely" be presented creating a $30 million medical school at WSU. The Wichita school would use mostly existing facilities and could not be ready before 1975 at the earliest. If the school were to build its own associated medical facilities, it would cost an additional $20 million.

There were, however, factors mitigating against a WSU full-fledged medical school. One was the pace of change in Kansas City. KUSM was developing a new curriculum on the modular system, was establishing a family practice department, was improving house officer training including increasing salaries for residents and interns, and had a definite schedule to increase the medical student classes to 250 by 1974. A second factor making it likely that Kansas City would be the focus of attention was cost. Expansion of the physical facilities at KUMC in Kansas City was a first priority. Reed said, "the hospital is in sad shape. They can't even continue at the 130-student level for long without better clinical facilities." It was unlikely that the state would fund a $30 million to $50 million school at Wichita while putting upwards of $50 million into expansion at Kansas City. The operating budget of KUMC was over $35 million, and it would probably cost $80 million a year to operate two Kansas medical schools. Reed pointed out, however, that many states did support two or more medical schools, and that the

Carnegie report concluded that communities over 350,000 in population should have a University Health Science Center. "Our immediate goal," he concluded, "should be to initiative dialogue regarding these matters, develop a position acceptable to MSSC, and then enlist full support from the community on that position." Pursuant to that, the board of the MSSC appointed an *ad hoc* committee for medical education.[80]

Reed was a diplomat. In his speeches early in 1971, he emphasized that it was appropriate to study a possible WSU medical school now, as developing one might have as much as a ten-year lead time. Certainly some legislators and planners could have been thinking of the WSU medical school as an inexpensive alternative to upgrading the Kansas City campus. Reed, however, did not push that line of thinking. It was not an "either/or" situation, he said, and Wichita would not seek its own medical school in preference to upgrading facilities at Kansas City.

While Reed said that Wichita was a "feasible location" for a medical school, he did not think it had to be an independent one with its own three- or four-year program, not to mention its own teaching hospital.[81] There had been delays in building new medical schools in Connecticut and in Massachusetts. In Kansas, educational expenditures generally had been frozen for fiscal year 1970–71, which might make huge spending on medical education seem particularly inappropriate. There would be a problem recruiting a "competent and willing faculty." Not only would there be the matter of recruiting faculty from elsewhere, but of attracting local physicians to full-time academic positions paying far less than they could and did make in private practice. In 1970, KUSM graduated 119 with a faculty of over 300.

A better alternative, Reed said, was a "community-based" school of medicine. This could be a campus "without walls" and, at first, without a large, full-time faculty. Students could come to Wichita only for their second two, clinical years and rotate through the several Wichita hospitals. They could be mentored and taught by a combination of part-time and volunteer faculty, who maintained their private practices and did not have regular academic appointments. There was even early thought of KU professors commuting to Wichita. WSU did have science departments, but had currently neither the staff nor the physical facilities to teach basic science to half of KU's medical students. Nor was that necessarily economical or desirable.[82] State representative Ervin Grant of El Dorado introduced a resolution in the spring of 1971 to consider WSU as the site of a second medical school. But Grant admitted he had not discussed it with Reed or WSU officials. "I don't know how they feel about it down there."[83] How they felt about it seemed to be evolving away from the political and fiscal long shot of establishing a second medical school and toward a community-based clinical program, perhaps closely coordinated with CHRP.

Dr. William Reals, who was president elect of the Medical Society of Sedgwick County, became visible in Wichita in 1971 on the same theme. Some sort of cooperative program with KUMC for Wichita would be a big enough step. The western two-thirds of Kansas would benefit a great deal, and it would mark the first time undergraduate medical students in Kansas would have been trained away from the Kansas/Missouri border area. Spreading the training geographically would help retention of doctors in the state: "If we expand the places people train, then we have a better chance of getting a hook on them." There had been approved advanced medical training programs in Wichita since World War II, and its hospitals and physicians were first rate. One hundred people were involved in residency and internship programs in Wichita and there were even four KU medical students getting their hospital training at Wichita hospitals on a voluntary basis because of certain specialties that were available there. It would be an easy and natural step simply to expand those programs.[84]

In June 1971, Wichita hosted representatives from 130 Kansas health-related schools to discuss a proposal for joint facilities, curriculum development, and perhaps shared faculty. The conference was coordinated by Dr. John Wong, associate dean and director of the Health Manpower Center at WSU, and was co-sponsored by WSU, the Kansas Regional Medical Program, and the Kansas Board of Health. While a Wichita medical school was not on the agenda, the conference further advertised the interest of Wichita and Wichita State in being a key player in statewide health education planning.[85]

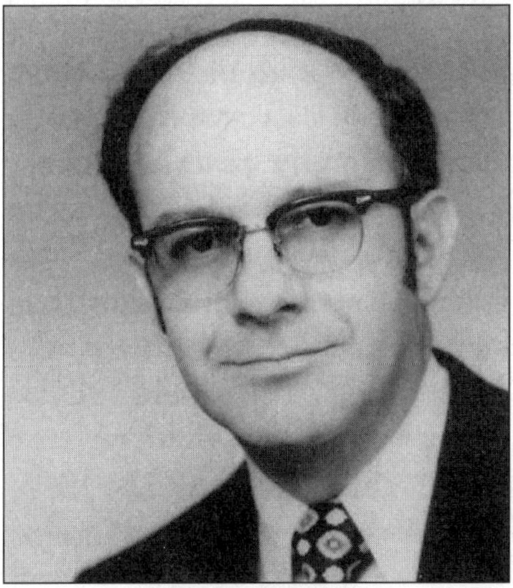
William Rieke, M.D.

Dr. William Rieke arrived in Kansas City in July to take over the reins at KUMC in the newly created post of Executive Vice Chancellor for Health Affairs. Rieke remembered that, at that point, both the University of Kansas and KUMC were in the "I'd like to see it happen" stage on many fronts. Rieke tried to put these together into a single and linked plan to present to the legislature. As Rieke saw it, the "three way deal" was that KUMC would increase the number in its undergraduate classes and residency programs significantly. Partly in order to do that, it would agree to a "branch" in Wichita where part of the expanded class would take its clinical training. But that would be tied to a major upgrade of the Kansas City facility funded by the state legislature.

Rieke made many trips to Wichita. He was impressed with Reed, and thought that Reed, who already had a joint appointment with WSU and KU, would be an ideal first dean for a Wichita community-based branch. Reed was a former Wichita physician with an outstanding reputation among his peers for integrity. He was also clearly a Wichitan with Wichita loyalties, and an alumnus of WSU to boot. And he had the confidence of President Ahlberg at WSU. In short, Reed might just be able to wear three hats—KU, WSU, and Wichita community—and coordinate those disparate interests in developing a Wichita branch of KUSM. Reed was a "fine person," Rieke thought, who had an easy way of working with people, and knew how to "look both ways" and include all those who needed including in planning and implementation. Also, he was a quiet worker who did not fly off the handle, get into personality wars with the charismatic, or "get too easily excited."[86]

Of course, it was a challenge for Rieke, too. He had experience in health centers in Washington and Iowa but he remembered that this "had not included even introductory training in the management of politics from a state that loved, hated, and continually publicized its medical center, or of a parent university thirty-five miles away that felt the same way about its medical branch in Kansas City." Rieke had no experience with medical "town-gown" problems "even remotely adequate to prepare me for the intense rivalries that existed in many non-academic practicing communities such as Johnson versus Sedgwick County or Kansas City versus Wichita." Yet, it was just those issues of coordinating the interest of state government, main and branch campuses, and external physicians and their medical organizations that he faced now. Rieke said he experienced a "steep and tumultuous learning curve" during the four years he was in office, not the least part of which involved the Wichita issue.[87]

That summer of 1971, alternatives floating around became a plan for presentation to the Board of Regents in the fall. Reed had written Walker in Kansas City in June: "I hate being so insistent about keeping informed regarding these matters; however, I have a great dread of continuing to espouse a concept down here that you may have abandoned. It's pretty hard to appear alert and well informed under the best of circumstances. Since I have to talk the line for two different 'shops,' I need to make certain that I don't promote misinformation in one area to the detriment of the other." Reed was being asked a lot of questions in Wichita. He said that if KUMC did not feel it could "hack an affiliation program at this time," he needed to change his speeches and "pull in some flags to keep from looking pretty silly."[88] In June, Reed's handwritten notes on a presentation to staff at St. Francis said: "Advocate letting Wichita be responsible for final two years. . . . If satisfactory answers from physicians then carefully study the necessary ingredients, money, etc. to participate as teaching center."[89]

Dr. E. Lawrence Chalmers, who replaced Clarke Wescoe as chancellor of the University of Kansas in 1969, had experience with cooperative programs in medicine, and thought this one could work. He thought Ahlberg of WSU "very much of a diplomat," and Reed a good implementer. "Wichita," Chalmers agreed, "needed and deserved some significant medical education in the community."[90] With Rieke's coordinated plan, in which he involved Reed, not only did the shape of a potential "clinical branch" in Wichita become more evident, but there was also a timetable for implementing what looked like a feasible project.

Rieke and Reed met with hospital officials in Wichita in July about some of the brass tacks. The hospital administrators were concerned whether there was an overall plan for regionalization of medical education in Kansas, whether KU would assist with the recruitment of Wichita faculty, whether the department chairs would be full-time and how they would be recruited, who would shoulder the cost of the residencies, how the concept of the chief of service being a KUMC clinical appointment would sell to the medical staff at the hospitals, and how the medical school "thing" would be finessed with the Medical Society of Sedgwick County and the CHRP advisory committee. It was clear that there was a plan for expanded medical education in Wichita, however many details remained to be worked out, including making sure that there was leadership in place.[91]

Also in July, Reed wrote Ahlberg asking the WSU president for his feelings about a planning document created by the KUMC administration concerning the suggested relationship of Reed, who was an associate dean at WSU and in charge of the CHRP program, with this new clinical branch project. There would be a meeting at KU in early August about the whole matter "at which time they will probably expect questions, not only from the hospital-community people but from us." Reed suggested that Ahlberg would probably share some of the concerns that he also had about the document, but that it was a good start.

Attached to Reed's letter was a document called "Draft for Discussion with Wichita Group." This was created by the dean and vice chancellor at KUMC with the input of the "ad hoc Committee for Affiliations" of KUMC, of which Reed was a member. It was a formal proposal for a "clinical branch" at Wichita to be developed in phases. When fully implemented, in about 1975, there would be two classes of fifty, 100 students total, in Wichita at all times. At the time, there was also a plan, implemented for a short time, to reduce the total medical school experience to three years, but this involved condensing the basic science core into an intensive eleven months rather than cutting the clinical years.

Some of the details concerned both Ahlberg and Reed because there seemed precious little autonomy or independence for the branch from KU or KUMC. There would be an advisory board for medical education formed in Wichita, and this board, together with the dean at KUSM and "with the advice and help of others at KU as desired and needed," would select an associate dean of KUSM "to be the dean's representative at the Wichita Clinical Branch." The department chairs at KUSM with advice from the advisory board and the associate dean would recruit full-time vice chairs of the Wichita departments, which the associate dean in Wichita would then appoint. These vice chairs would have to ask the department chairs at Kansas City for approval of many of their actions. For the first several years, each salaried faculty in Wichita would be expected to spend a two-week period in residence at KUMC in his or her own discipline. Faculty from Kansas City could rotate through Wichita and the branch could have one Kansas City faculty always in residence. All professional fees would go into a Wichita Medical Education Fund to be administered by the KU Endowment Association. This money would be spent at the initiative of the Wichita department vice chairs and with the approval of the chairs and dean in Kansas City, unless the dean in Kansas City delegated this to the associate dean in Wichita.[92]

That did not exactly give Wichita peer status. Rieke well understood that, but understood as well the concerns at Lawrence and Kansas City about the dangers of too much independence for Wichita—concerns that could sink the whole project. He understood that WSU had an interest in being the administrator of the branch and of the hospital residency programs, too. However, he thought it was important to keep the channel of funding and decision-making running through the University of Kansas. Partly this was "company loyalty," but partly it turned on the need for Wichita's accreditation through the only university in the state with a strong existing health education program.

Nothing in that thinking prevented responding to change in the future. Rieke and Reed had many conversations about CHRP perhaps one day teaching more basic science, and the branch perhaps someday evolving into a four-year institution. Rieke recalled later, "Cramer would have been pleased with that and I could have been pleased with that." But in 1971, Rieke was understandably concerned both with the personal and institutional politics and with the problem of dilution that was raised by the minimal overall budget from the state legislature. As it was, precious little, he thought, was going to KUMC to maintain quality. He did not want to be responsible for a dilution of that quality by moving too quickly or too far in a crisis mode. Perhaps the legislature would have been satisfied with something more "slipshod and easier" Rieke surmised, but it was his job to educate them and the public about what good medical education really was.

Wichita's community-based branch would be a different kind of institution than KUMC. It would have a different mission, and it would be "freed in a sense" by less need to earn tenure, to do research, to publish, and to be promoted through full-time academic ranks. But it had to be taken seriously. Rieke knew that neither Wichita nor its physicians would like to be considered second rate or, worse, actually to be a second rate institution. It, of course, had to be accredited, and accredited in coordination with KUSM. "It had to be real," he remembered, "could not be contrived." His administrative style was to find good people to run things in Wichita and then "hold an umbrella over them so they don't get rained on."[93] He started with Dr. Cramer Reed.

Legislative action proceeded. There were two concurrent house resolutions (1054 and 1032) in the spring of 1971 concerning the Wichita branch. The first, passed in March, established a joint legislative committee to study existing facilities in Kansas for the education of physicians and physician assistants and "to prepare a plan which will expand such opportunities for education within the state." The second established another committee to "make a comprehensive study of the establishment of a medical school within Wichita State University. The committee shall study and report upon the cost of equipping and operating such a medical school and all other fiscal needs with special emphasis upon the cost of the first year of operation." This course of action was not recommended by the Regents, but was pushed by some legislators.[94]

Wichita pushed it, too. A resolution of the Board of Commissioners of the City of Wichita dated June 22, 1971, established an *ad hoc* committee called the Medical School Advisory Committee. This was to study and advise the city "on the feasibility and potential of developing the concept of a local medical school, utilizing the resources, financial or otherwise, of local state and federal agencies."[95] Early in July the committee met, with Robert Gadberry of the Fourth National Bank as chair and Drs. James Donnell of the City Commission, William Swisher of the

Medical Society of Sedgwick County, George Lappin of the Wichita VA Hospital, and Dr. William Reals as members. Reals said he did not "see this in any way as a threat to KU Medical Center and the effort may tie nicely into KUMC's hope to expand the last two years of medical education to Wichita."[96] However, when representatives of the American Medical Association were invited to Wichita to discuss a school of medicine, and when Dr. Donnell visited Washington to seek independent funding at the White House level, no doubt it ruffled some feathers at KUMC.[97]

Early in September 1971, the medical center committee of the Kansas Board of Regents met in the boardroom at Morrison Hall on the WSU campus. President Ahlberg described discussions between himself and Wolf over the last several years concerning cooperative plans for health education, and he distributed his December 1969 letter concerning the basis for such cooperation and the sharing of control and pay of Dr. Reed. Dr. Rieke spoke to a similar theme, saying that all were agreed "as far as the concept is concerned," to place a certain number of medical students at Wichita for two or three years of training and to expand the graduate training of house officers in Wichita. Rieke also stated that all were agreed that course should be taken "rather than to work for a separate medical school at Wichita." There followed "considerable discussion," at the end of which a plan was approved. Reed and Ahlberg spoke of the problems WSU faced as the result of inadequate legislative funding for CHRP and felt that, if the program remained weak, the cooperative program for medical students would seem "unrealistic in the eyes of the faculty and medical people in Wichita." The Regents agreed to take up that question at their regular September meeting along with the whole issue of establishing a cooperative clinical branch of KUSM at Wichita. Ahlberg agreed to make arrangements for a dinner meeting with the Wichita press.[98]

At their September 17, 1971 meeting in Pittsburg, Kansas, the Kansas Board of Regents approved the Wichita clinical branch of KUSM. Reed became the dean while continuing as dean of the WSU College of Health Related Professions. The first students were to start at Wichita in the fall of 1973.[99] Dr. Rieke commented to the student newspaper at the University of Kansas, "It's the most significant development in medical education in Kansas in the last fifty years."[100]

Chapter Three
Going Forth

Nearly everyone involved with the new KU clinical branch in Wichita agreed on one thing, namely that Dr. Cramer Reed seemed to be the right person to pull all the disparate factions together. His "leadership, vision, drive, and commitment" was a thing often commented upon. "He knew the community and the community knew him," commented Dwight Allen, executive director of the Medical Society of Sedgwick County.[101] A classmate of Reed's at Washington University Medical School of St. Louis noted that his friend "gets along with everybody and has a way of making you feel good," but "on the other hand I think he was pretty determined on these things."[102] Dr. Ernest Crow, who became the first chair of internal medicine at the Wichita school said, "I don't know where Cramer got all those ideas, but most of them were good."[103] Some of Reed's ideas, such as coordinating CHRP with the clinical branch to train the medical teams he foresaw in the future, did not advance much. Others, like the humanizing of medical education, and the enormous outreach he envisioned across the western part of the state, did not work as well as he wished. But he was instrumental in recruiting the faculty, establishing the Wichita unit, and gaining its acceptance as something both legitimate and permanent. He bridged the gaps between Wichita State, KU, the Wichita medical community, KUMC, and the state legislature, not to mention holding together an early medical faculty in Wichita of unprecedented range, background, income, and variety of current interests. The explanation always by those observing was that, while the school in Wichita was not exactly the shadow of one man in an Emersonian sense, it came close. Reed's personality and aims set the tone and the direction.

Reed himself was an unselfish builder, a tireless worker, and a charismatic, though quiet leader. Maysel White remembered Reed was "a giant in his field and much beloved. I don't know if the word is fury but it is close. . . . He was the glue and it [the Wichita branch] was a vision of his."[104] Dr. Dean Kortge, a Ph.D. in history who doubtless never would have found a place in a more traditional medical school organization, noted that Reed could appeal to altruism "because he lived it. . . . Not many people live their life like Cramer Reed."[105] He could also appeal to Wichita pride because he lived that too. And he related to the students who eventually started coming to Wichita from the Kansas City campus like no dean they had ever experienced. Dr. Garold Minns, who eventually became associate dean at Wichita himself, was in the second class in Wichita, and was impressed by the strong collegiality between residents, students, and faculty, with Reed maintaining the atmosphere. Reed would take time to sit and chat with students, giving them the feeling that the hierarchy was only an accident of age and experience. They were led by Reed to believe they were colleagues with faculty and staff at Wichita, the only distinction being that they were earlier in their training than their mentors.[106] Reed was a person who became powerful by not acting powerful, and he created a fierce loyalty through his extraordinary people skills. Dr. George Farha, a Wichita surgeon and first department head of surgery at Wichita called Cramer Reed "a gentleman's gentleman."[107] Marlin Rein, who had a strong suspicion of Wichita's ambition, still much admired its dean. Reed was, he said, "a sweetheart of a guy."[108] Reed was, Dr. Fred Sudermann of WSU remembered, "the perfect guy for the job," although the job eventually may have gotten too big for anyone.[109] That it was big from the start, both heavyweight and delicate of execution, Reed and his small staff learned soon enough.

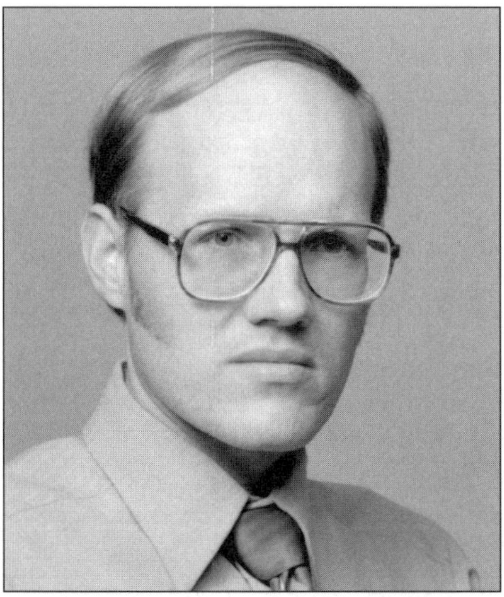

Garold Minns, M.D. and Associate Dean, was in the second graduating class at KUSM-W.

Physically, the early school in Wichita seemed nearly invisible. The new operation was housed in a two-bedroom house across from the Newman Center at 17th and Roosevelt on the WSU campus—"a modest place for the dean of a medical school to be" one physician

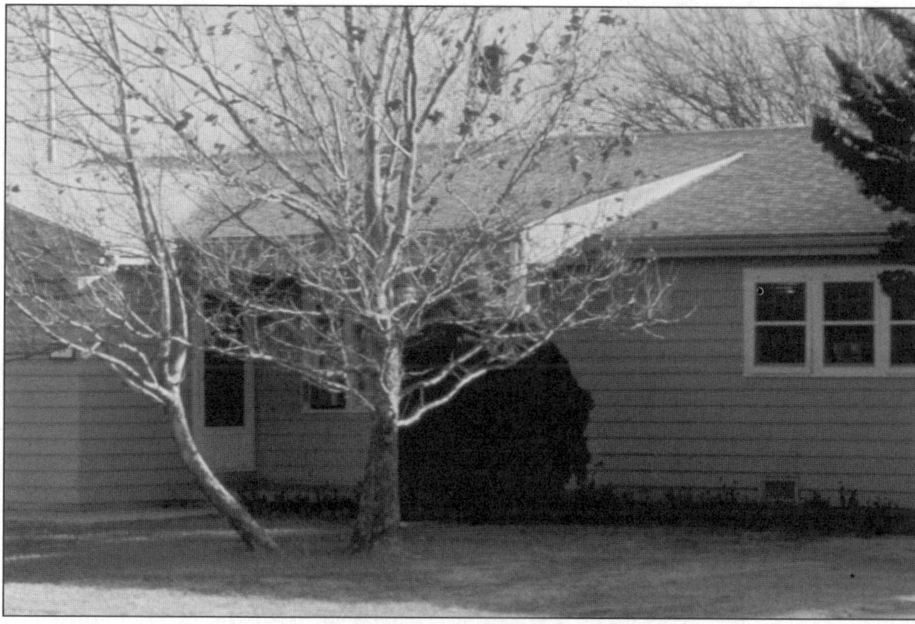

House on 17th Street, KUSM-W's first home.

thought.[110] Hazel Fenske, part of that staff, was over fifty at the time and looking for work because her husband had been dismissed at Boeing. She was typical of the kind of non-traditional employee whose potential Reed could see. She went a block to make copies, arranged for the staff at the Wichita branch to share a bathroom in another house, and shortly became the best friend and tireless champion of the Wichita medical students—"kind of like a grandma to them." Little did she imagine at the time that eventually she would have a room named after her at a large and modern facility "and I did not even have to die,"[111] she said. It was all modest, even miniscule with none of the administrative trappings associated with a major, or even a minor, institution for medical training.

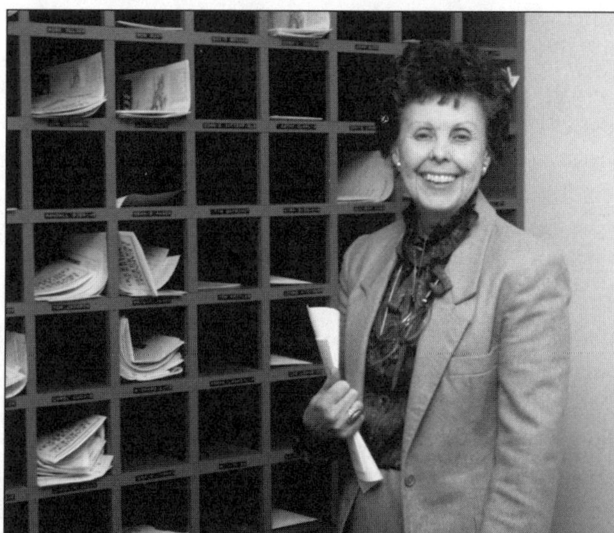

Early staff member, Hazel Fenske.

But the "Wichita Branch" was the acorn from which a spreading oak might grow and people all over the state were aware of that. Therefore controversy swirled around it and around what were seen by its enemies, despite its obvious low profile, as its pretensions.

Central to the complaints was the thought that Wichita and/or Wichita State University would use the branch as the entering wedge for empire building in medical education. Certainly there were some in town who had that in mind. The *Wichita Beacon* reported in September 1971, as the Wichita school was authorized, "There seems to be more misunderstanding than accord at the moment." The plan had been approved by the directors of the Medical Society of Sedgwick County, not by the full membership, and the reporter thought there were some "hard feelings there." Some in town, the article went on, would like to see a full-fledged medical school in Wichita "and the day probably will come when that will be an actuality," but for the present it would be best to cooperate with the KU initiative. Dr. James Donnell, a Wichita city commissioner, made no secret of his interest in a separate school. He said, "The easy way to get a medical school in Wichita is to work with KU."[112] Expanding on that thought, he added, "I think we're on our way to having a medical school. It may be a branch of KU but, as I would see it, would be a three- or four-year curricular medical school." He thought such a school would be "virtually autonomous" in relation to KUMC and would eventually have both basic science and clinical components. Dr. Ernest Crow, representing the Medical Society added that many physicians in town saw the branch as a first step toward a full medical school in the city.[113]

Outside Wichita, that sort of talk was anathema. The *Salina Journal* commented that no sooner had plans for a clinical branch gotten underway than "the Hot Air Capital got busy. . . . Sedgwick County physicians took pot shots at KU and at each other and a glorious dream was had by all." Wichita had pushed for a state university of its own and now it wanted its own medical school. Whitley Austin, the editor at Salina, thought the result would be that "the rest of us pay for the miracle" in Wichita. Never, he thought, could Wichita be satisfied to be a subordinate, "not with its political clout, not with its burning and parochial ambitions." Kansas, Austin thought, did not need "more tax-eating monuments to metropolitan pride."[114] The *Lawrence Daily Journal-World* chimed in. KUMC was having trouble making ends meet financially as it was. A satellite branch was okay, but another medical school was not. How could Wichita create the physical facilities, much less the faculty for a first class medical school? "There may be a number of doctors in Wichita who would like to be able to say, 'Yes, I'm on the staff at the Wichita medical school,' but do these doctors have the ability to give a quality medical education to young men and women," the paper read. The view from Lawrence was that an independent Wichita medical school would be a second-class school. "Would a topflight prospective medical student be quite so interested in obtaining his medical education in Kansas if he had justifiable reason to wonder where he might be assigned for his education, Wichita or Kansas City?"[115] Yes, some had said it would be a bargain. A $20 million science building could be built at Wichita with 75 percent federal funding. But, wrote the *Russell Record*, "there's a whole can of worms to be sorted out before legislators can afford the luxury of another medical school, particularly when taxpayers are being billed—and students short-changed."[116] If the existing Kansas higher education was hurting, wrote the *Emporia Gazette*, "what will happen when the Wichita School of Medicine gets its bite?"[117]

However bitter was the invective against Wichita ambition and the thought of an independent medical school, there was a good deal of support around the state for the present concept of a community-based clinical branch at Wichita controlled by KUMC. Governor Robert Docking supported the Wichita plan as one that would encourage doctors to stay in Kansas and train them "in one of the most inexpensive methods known." It would bring Wichita's hospitals "an additional influx of sophisticated men and women and equipment enhancing its resources for quality medical care," while increasing WSU's "department of educational resources for students interested in basic sciences."[118] Clyde Reed, the powerful editor of the *Parsons Sun*, and no friend of Wichita generally, called the plan "feasible and economical." The editor at Chanute felt good about the hospital facilities in Wichita, the doctors there, he thought, would be more student-oriented and care-oriented than research-oriented, and the possibility that more family practice doctors interested in practicing in small towns would emerge. "For the first time," he wrote, "a sizeable number of Kansas physicians will find themselves supporting a program not to the liking of their alma mater."[119] In fact, insofar as those physicians were represented by the Kansas Medical Society, they did approve. Dr. William Reals, president of the medical society, praised the Wichita plan.[120] A ballot taken at KUMC showed that "most" faculty there supported it. Executive Vice Chancellor Rieke stated, "This branch will provide for a new emphasis and better balance in medical education as well as for increased production."[121]

The infant branch in Wichita, that fall of 1971, was characterized by the local newspaper as an "iffy" proposition. It had plenty of enemies and only one year's funding. If—and only if—the 1972 legislature approved the linked and expensive renovation program at Kansas City would it be likely either that KUSM would carry out the expansion of its class or that it would continue to plan on sending students to Wichita. "Dr. Reed," the press reported, "takes all of the money trouble with equal mixtures of optimism and caution." He was, the reporter said, "a man growing accustomed to such problems." There would be the advantage that Wichita physicians would initially have a good deal of autonomy in creating the administrative style and the curriculum for the Wichita school. Reed planned to build on some planning groups that had existed in town to create an advisory group both to receive gifts and to generate legislative support.[122] In December, KU Chancellor E. Lawrence Chalmers and WSU President Clark Ahlberg recommended that the regents authorize Rieke and Reed to develop a table of organization and guidelines for the administration of the branch.[123] As a start on public relations, Reed, Don Granger of the *Eagle*, Roy House of Wesley Hospital, and Donald Conroy of St. Francis Hospital appeared on KTVH-TV in Wichita to discuss the topic "More Doctors for Kansas."[124]

Dr. Rieke, for one, was positive both that the KUMC expansion would be funded, that the Wichita connection would remain, and that it would thrive to the benefit of KUMC as well as Wichita hospitals and doctors. He wrote the entering freshman class at KUSM late in 1971, "These are challenging and exciting times for medical schools and their students. Many new and different plans for securing a medical education are being tested in various schools across the nation." The branch at Wichita was a good model and "we are now working diligently with the Wichita community and Wichita State University to accomplish this." There would be only a small number assigned to Wichita at first—sixteen in the initial class in 1973, so "the probability of your being involved is remote," but it was only fair to inform applicants of the possibility.[125]

There was another crucial step involved, namely the funding for the KUMC expansion in Kansas City. Dr. Rieke was determined that this be included in the expansion in Wichita, the decentralized hospital-based residency programs around the state, the outreach in other parts of the state, and the new emphasis on family practice. Clifford Griffin was just finishing his substantial history of the University of Kansas, published in 1974, and in 1972 there was a new chancellor in Lawrence, Dr. Archie Dykes. Dykes was both a hard driving hands-on manager and a strong proponent of the "one university" concept. With all the tradition behind it that its history reflected, and with the strong alumni group that supported it financially and politically, Dykes and Rieke thought the early 1970s was a poor time to have the University of Kansas splintering. KUMC itself would have to continue to be an integral part of the University of Kansas centered at Lawrence, even though, by now, all its direct facilities were located in Kansas City, and the same would need to be true of the Wichita campus. Dykes felt that the Wichita extension of KUSM could be very strengthening for KUMC and for KU in the sense that it caused the state line medical school to be "more deeply imbedded in the state."[126] But it would have to be clear that it was part of KU, not a separate empire. "We knew where we wanted to go," remembered Patricia Head, who had responsibility for the KU alumni organization, "but just had to get there."[127]

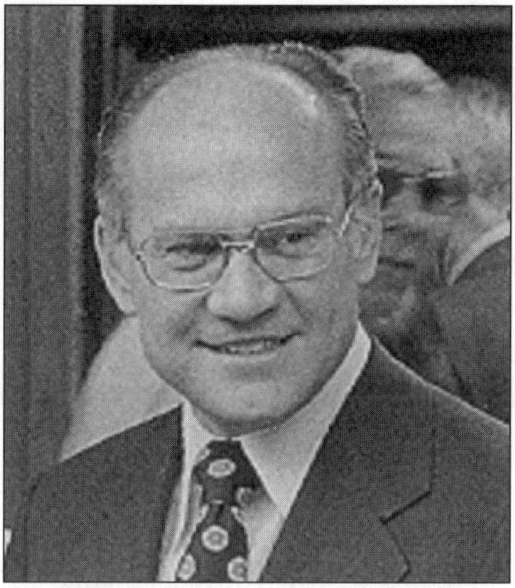

Chancellor Archie Dykes

There was considerable lobbying in Topeka in 1972 about the funding for KUMC, which was, after all, one of the major single investments in physical plant the state legislature had ever made. The price was escalating fast in the inflationary economy of the 1970s and, by the time the expansion got the approval of the legislature in March 1972, the price tag was nearly $65 million.[128] At the same time the curriculum was reduced (it turned out for a short time only) to three years, something that had been tried briefly in World War II and would again prove a temporary way to save time and money.[129] Old buildings at Goat Hill, the first home in Kansas City for the KU School of Medicine when three private hospitals had consolidated to form it in 1906, were torn down at the same time. It had not served as a hospital for many years, and the campus of KUMC had long ago moved, but still it was symbolic of the jettisoning of the past and the transition to the future with KUMC and what had been for it an unwilling exercise in historic preservation in a high-tech world.[130]

Reed thought that the debates could be the end of the Wichita initiative. He wrote Dr. Russell Nelson, a pediatrician involved with the Wesley residency program: "It appears that we are presently confronted with a temporary hiatus in terms of meaningful progress toward fully activating the Wichita State Branch of the University of Kansas School of Medicine, until such time as it is ascertained whether or not the legislature will recommend funding of the fiscal year 1973 program. Be that as it may, I hope you will not be deterred in your efforts to establish a community-based pediatric residency and/or inception of a relationship with the Department of Pediatrics at the University of Kansas School of Medicine." Regardless of how the Wichita clinical branch project might fare in the budget, Reed wrote, "it appears that the concept of providing elective clinical clerkship opportunities in the Wichita community hospital system is one that should be encouraged for several reasons quite unrelated to any undergraduate student involvement."[131]

The 1972 debates created another opportunity both for proponents of a wider role for Wichita and for opponents of any role for Wichita to criticize the plan for the branch as presented. Dolph Simons, Jr. in the *Lawrence Journal* brought up the specter of duplication again and of diminution of quality. The expansion of Kansas City would cost enough, he wrote, and "regardless of the cost, what kind of excellence can be offered to the students in a split medical school setup? . . . How long will it be before Wichita promoters start calling for a state supported law school?" What had happened to the original idea that WSU would be supervised by KU? "Many in Wichita talk openly of the time when Wichita will be the largest school in the state system, giving orders to the other, smaller institutions at Lawrence and Manhattan."[132] The *Russell Daily News* editor said that schools all over the state were "straining with status-seeking enthusiasm." Emporia did not want to be called a teacher's college anymore, and every institution wanted to be called a university. "Efforts of Wichita now underway to sneak a medical college through the legislature at the expense of the University of Kansas Medical School in Kansas City is typical. Wichita State University, a gift to the state a few years ago, is what can happen when politicians and educators are given a free hand."[133] There was nothing inevitable about Wichita imposing its will, but inviting that large, industrial city to the party, seemed to other towns, rather like welcoming a bull into a china shop.

And despite Reed's diplomatic, low-key approach, sometimes Wichita did indeed act a bit like a bull. One source of this was community ambition. Another was institutional ambition at Wichita State.

The community pressure arose, in part, through doctors, though the medical community was definitely split on the issue. Dr. Lew Purinton, for example, supported the branch, but thought the idea of a four-year medical school for Wichita was an impractical one.[134] However, Dr. William McGuire, a Wichita pediatrician, disagreed, and joined Dr. Donnell in promoting the idea that the branch might be only a first step. McGuire wrote the *Wichita Eagle* early in 1972 that Wichita had a "progressive, every-moving university," and a full complement of doctors, labs and hospitals. It even had a large vacant hotel that, in a distressed economy, needed a use. McGuire thought the $60 million plus being spent in Kansas City would be better spent in Wichita, and he seriously proposed that a four-year Wichita medical school be considered as an alternative to that funding.[135] McGuire corresponded with Reed about it and also with Max Bickford, the executive of the Kansas Board of Regents, on this subject. Reed was conciliatory, but firm. He appreciated McGuire's concern "as a fellow Wichitan," he wrote, but Reed's position as a state employee "does not permit me to make any broad, sweeping or grandiose statements now (or at any time, for that matter), but I simply must solicit your indulgence and understanding of the situation." Reed intimated, that the expansion at Kansas City, far from being a threat to Wichita's future in medical education, was the *sine qua non*, for it having any future in that field at all. And once the furor died down, there was a good chance that the local future would be bright. Reed would be glad to sit down and talk with McGuire "to acquaint you with some facts that are not apparent on the surface."[136]

Another source of community push was businesspeople. The Wichita Chamber of Commerce had contacted WSU President Ahlberg and Dean Reed late in 1971, asking: "What is the status and likelihood of developing a medical school in Wichita? Should this come to fruition would it mean that there would be greater physician availability throughout Kansas?"[137] Monte Johnson, vice president of the Fourth National Bank and Trust Company in Wichita wrote Reed: "I can't think of any phase of the University that is receiving more meaningful publicity than is the College of Health Related Professions. With your dynamic leadership I wouldn't be surprised if they switched the entire medical school operation from Kansas City to Wichita someday."[138] Another strong business supporter was Larry Jones, president of the Coleman Company. Jones was part of a group of businesspeople that contributed time and money to the Wichita branch with the hope that it might become an independent medical school, but certainly with the expectation that it would be closely connected with WSU and enhance that local institution considerably. The community, Jones stated a few years later, had struggled to get WSU into the state system. It "rose up as a unified force to embrace the University, to advance its cause, and to exercise its latent leadership and political muscle. Few times before or since has this happened. Thus, the university is an historic monument, a symbol, or rather proud creature of the community." There would be no Wichita branch of KUSM at all, Jones thought, had it not been "nourished and advanced by Wichitans against a negative state environment." These backers would be disturbed if they perceived that KU had quashed or unduly controlled it without a proper consideration of local views and interests.[139]

Indeed what role WSU was to play was, and remained for some time, a central question concerning the future of the Wichita operation of KUSM. It was obvious that initially there was some connection. CHRP had been started as a joint project. The branch was physically housed on the WSU campus for some years—first in the little house, then at Fairmount Towers, a WSU dormitory, and finally, at least in drawings and

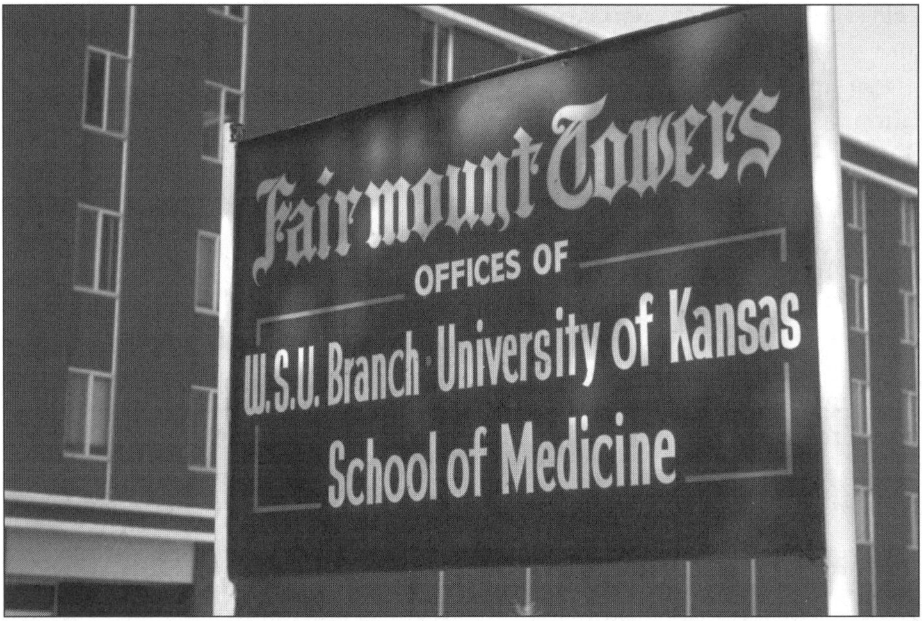

Fairmount Towers

plans, in a new building on the campus that was to house both CHRP and the school of medicine. Once the naming process went beyond the casual reference to the place as the "branch," the first official name on the stationery was "The Wichita State University Branch of the University of Kansas School of Medicine."[140] Reed made the point regularly in fact that "one great basic difference existing in this community from the very beginning, is the fact that the 'idea' of Wichita becoming the base of a community medical education effort did not evolve from any local ground swell. It was literally proposed by KU and Wichita State, and thus continues to be subject to some scrutiny."[141] In fact, according to Reed and consultants who visited, there existed in Wichita a "University takeover syndrome."[140] That is, both hospitals and chamber of commerce boosters were concerned lest the vehicle become too dominant. That was the ancient "town-gown" suspicion with which every educational institution had always had to dwell.

Reed, characteristically, downplayed the WSU connection while not denying it or criticizing it. Yes, Ahlberg had had some conversations with state legislators, perhaps even had gone to the point of making estimates for a building on the WSU campus to house the branch. Perhaps this meant to him that a brand new school was being considered. Reed said later he was not sure he knew "how Clark felt about it." But it was clear that Ahlberg was more assertive about WSU's role than was Reed, who was trying to salvage the project itself for the town, however it was administered. Reed remembered that there was a meeting in the Morrison Hall boardroom at WSU once where the subject was what to call the new Wichita branch. Ahlberg suggested calling it the Wichita State University Branch of the University of Kansas School of Medicine. While Reed did not think that sat well with the KU people, nevertheless, that name was used for a time.[143]

KU representatives understood WSU's interest, and saw possibilities for joint administration, but feared that the lion and the lamb might not be able to co-exist peaceably. Reed was in the middle, trying to balance community interests and ambitions, those of KU and KUMC and those of the hospitals. Reed thought Chancellor Dykes understood the need for some autonomy for the branch. "He may not have felt that way, but acted that way," is how Reed put it. And he thought Rieke understood very well that certainly in the initial recruiting and development of curriculum and mission the best way to use Reed's talents was to give him a little room to operate.[144]

But the presence of rival WSU in the mix complicated the issue for the KU people. There was, Dykes remembered later, a "healthy tension" between the two institutions about into whose jurisdiction the new branch should fall. "It was a very important undertaking for the Kansas legislature." It had high visibility and a high priority. Ahlberg and Dykes had a number of conversations about it. Dykes respected Ahlberg and thought him a "fabulously successful university president," but understood that his and Ahlberg's interests here were different, and that Ahlberg naturally acted as an "able proponent" for WSU. There were models in other states for decentralization of medical education, but neither Dykes nor Governor Robert Docking wanted that to happen in Kansas. Dykes thought that what Kansas did "in retrospect may have been a very wise decision."

There was division among state legislators, however. State Senator Wesley Sowers acted as a strong proponent for more of a Wichita and WSU role.[145] But the Sedgwick County delegation in general was not strong in the legislative leadership. Marlin Rein, who began working with the legislative research department and state budget office in 1973, remembered not only sharing some cold ham sandwiches with Reed, but also "correcting" the language of both Reed and Ahlberg when talking about the WSU School of Medicine. "He would talk about his medical school," Rein remembered of conversations with Ahlberg. "He never had a medical school." And there were no doubt other discussions—"who knows what was said." Rein understood there "was a high sense of ownership of the school in Wichita," and said that some of its struggles to cement that were "painful to watch." There were issues, he thought, that went far beyond medical education. Even the seemingly straightforward question of where to house the Wichita clinical branch caused political and economic struggles from the very beginning, with local hospitals maneuvering to provide the facility, and with WSU and the state legislature eventually splitting on that question after a period of cooperation. These matters made the first years of growth of the medical school in Wichita "times that tried every man's soul."[146] The ultimate outcome was anything but certain in 1972.

Both Dykes and Ahlberg were aware that Reed was trying to serve two masters, and that, as Dykes was to put it, there was "inherent in the role he was playing a fairly large amount of frustration."[147] The masters were, John Breazeale from WSU remembered, "not at war, but not peaceful either." The Wichita program was the "political hot potato in the state at the time" with "overt and outspoken opponents," and therefore Breazeale was most impressed that Reed kept all the balls in the air. Perhaps, Breazeale thought, the troubles Chancellor Chalmers had with student protest on civil rights at a surprisingly radical KU campus in some ways protected the Wichita medical education program from some of the not always welcome attention it might otherwise have received from Lawrence.[148]

At any rate Reed immediately took the reins and advanced the program once the last strategic hurdle was cleared with the funding of the KUMC expansion. Rieke worked with Roger Lowe at WSU on Reed's salary. He was 100 percent on the KU payroll from April to June 1972 and then 50 percent KU and 50 percent WSU.[149] He had been studying models of divided medical schools in other states, and he intensified this in 1972. Among the inquiries were to Kent State, the Tulsa branch of the Oklahoma medical school, an interinstitutional agreement between Indiana University and Purdue for medical education in Indiana, the Southern Illinois University School of Medicine at Springfield, Illinois, and the Rockford School of Medicine, also in Illinois.[150] Surprisingly, he found that these schools were often as interested in the ideas being developed at Wichita as he was in mining their experience.[151]

The whole concept was new and Wichita was on the leading edge of it. But it was a trend with legs. By 2003 twenty-five of the nation's medical schools had at least two campuses, the second of which was customarily a regional clinical campus like the one that started in Wichita in the early 1970s. Twenty-four such branches were founded in the period 1970–1975, far more than in any similar period since. Many cities that had been identified in the 1970 Carnegie report as prime sites for medical schools became, as did Wichita, the locus for a clinical "branch" campus tied to the main medical school in the state. The creation of most of them, as in Wichita, was driven by the expansion of graduate medical education around the country and the need for hospital-based residency programs to have some association with a university school of medicine. There was often also the recognition, as in Wichita, that the increased patient base in an urban center with strong community hospitals might be an advantage to the main medical school. On the other hand, the community where the branch was located would likely benefit by being better able to recruit specialists to the area.[152] Wichita, which was so typical of all this, became an "incubator" in a sense where some gained experience who were later to administer such schools in other parts of the nation.[153]

People on other campuses, whom Reed contacted between 1971 and 1973 when he was researching the field intensively, understood both the promise and the risks of the creation of such "secondary" clinical branches. "There is no doubt in my mind," wrote Dr. Richard Moy, dean at Southern Illinois, "that the school will be judged on the basis of far more than its output of physician manpower." It must be involved in allied health education, continuing education, and the health care delivery system itself. It should also enhance the professional life of doctors in its region, "hold and attract health talent" and "rationalize health care and improve its quality." It was a tall order. But Moy concluded, "I have the distinct feeling that if the people of our area are not receiving more and better health care by the end of the decade we will be harshly judged."[154] No doubt Reed had that "distinct feeling" also. One of his firm convictions, shared with Moy and others on the front lines of the community-based medical school movement, was that a modern physician must be not only a great healer but a "complete citizen," aware of the circumstances that were creating social turbulence. The doctor should be willing and able to be a leader in public health matters in the community.[155]

The administrative details began to emerge along with the features that would make what was eventually to be called the University of Kansas School of Medicine-Wichita (KUSM-W) unique.[156] Rieke, in

October 1972, made a list of "understandings," arrived at in discussions with Reed. Even though it fit the mission that there would be large numbers of part-time and volunteer faculty, it would be policy that each clinical discipline would eventually have at least one, preferably more, full-time faculty members. There would be no rigidity about holding Wichita faculty salaries absolutely in line with Kansas City. In fact, Wichita full-time salaries might have to be higher in the initial absence of clinical income for academic faculty. The departments at Wichita were to be administratively autonomous from KUSM departments except for formal lines from the departments to Reed and from Reed to Rieke. The two agreed also, even this early, that the physical location at WSU might prove awkward in defining the real relationship between KU and WSU regarding the new facility. "It would be most desirable," Rieke wrote, "for us to pursue a 'neutral' specifically identifiable home base for the WSU branch." The Sedgwick County Hospital, located west of WSU on Ninth Street, was a suggestion. Since the institution of Medicare and Medicaid in the mid-1960s, its patient base had declined drastically, and it might be a facility the county would be more than willing to sell. "I understand your reluctance to admit acute care patients in such a facility immediately," Rieke wrote, "but hope that this possibility to establish a teaching base 'at home' isn't forgotten for the future." He reserved $258,500 for Reed to spend in fiscal year 1972–73 for house staff stipends and other purposes.[157]

All the while Rieke tried to emphasize—to McDill "Huck" Boyd, to Wes Sowers, and to others in the legislature—that Wichita was part of a package. "I emphasize . . . the need for *togetherness* and not geographic factionalism in our program. What we are doing is for the good of all Kansas."[158] Reed was speaking the same language in talks and in letters. In February 1973, he responded to an editorial by Clyde Reed referring to the new Wichita branch as the "Chamber of Commerce Medical School." He emphasized that the reference to the WSU branch in a recent house bill as "the Wichita State University Medical Center" did not reflect the official posture of its administration.[159] There was, he said, "absolutely no dichotomy of opinion on the part of President Ahlberg or myself regarding the propriety of Kansas supporting only one medical center of which we are pleased to be a viable component."[160] Rieke spoke in Wichita and Reed attended meetings in Kansas City. When Dykes became chancellor at KU, he was a regular visitor to Wichita also. The local newspaper agreed that "the program can never work if an atmosphere of suspicion and parochialism exists."[161] And all connected with it wanted it to work.

In July 1972, KUSM-W received its first faculty member, Dr. G. Gayle Stephens, who became chair of the Department of Family Practice.[162] This was one of nine, full-time, paid positions funded and for which the school was authorized to recruit in anticipation of students arriving within a year. Philosophy and politics were about to hit the ground and become educational practice.

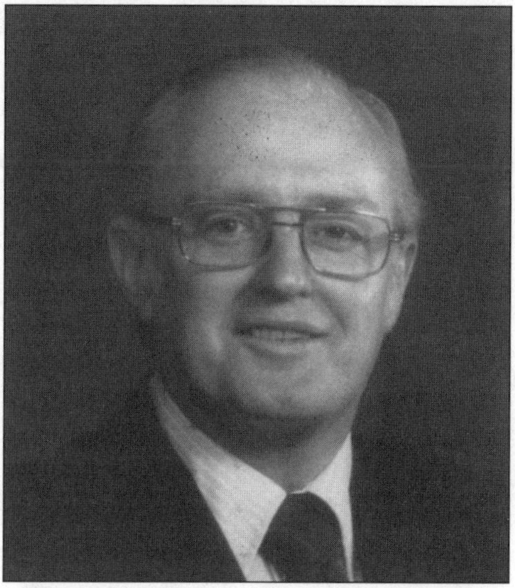

G. Gayle Stephens, M.D., first faculty member and Chair of the Department of Family Practice.

Chapter Four
PEOPLING THE PLAN

Dr. Cramer Reed sat down in the late summer of 1972 for an interview with *Wichita Eagle* columnist Don Granger about "a program quietly developing in two frame cottages on the campus of Wichita State University." One of these houses, a green ranch style at 1821 North Roosevelt was headquarters for the WSU College of Health Related Professions and the other, a low gray ranch at 3720 East 17th, was for KUSM-W. It appeared then that the WSU connection would remain strong. Not only was the official name still the Wichita State University Branch of the University of Kansas School of Medicine, but the planning was for its administrative offices to move eventually into a new Life Science Building that was in the campus development plan.

Reed waxed enthusiastic. Community hospitals, he said, were "where the action is, where 'real' medicine is practiced, where 'relevance prevails'," and therefore the "community-based" feature of KUSM-W was exciting. Various states had established satellite schools, a few freestanding separate medical schools. "The WSU Branch of KUSM," Reed said, "is a variation on this theme, and is subject to all the assorted pressures and controversy as well as making a major contribution to the improved health of all Kansans." He envisioned the future of medicine in the team concept combining the skills of the doctor with the medical support of students trained by CHRP. Instead of a doctor and nurse, as in the early days, there might be a doctor and seven paraprofessionals on a team. While there was no direct administrative relationship, other than Reed himself, linking KUSM-W and WSU's CHRP, Reed thought the interrelationship of the two schools was "logical and inescapable." Most of the medical faculty at KUSM-W would, he thought, have joint appointments at CHRP. He would offer teaching positions on a volunteer and part-time basis to all members of the Medical Society of Sedgwick County. "We want very much to rediscover the value of the practicing physician in the teaching of medicine. He (or she) should, if he so desires, be restored to his rightful place as a first-class citizen in the world of academic medicine." Each doctor who volunteered as a teacher of medical students would get exactly the same reward, "the unpaid satisfaction of discharging a duty to medicine and the community." There would, of course, be department heads, and full- and part-time paid faculty would fill out the complement. Graduate education in close cooperation with the hospitals would also develop. The Wichita Medical Education Association (which later became the Wichita Center for Graduate Medical Education, or WCGME) had been formed in June 1972, with Roy House, Wesley Hospital's chief administrator, at its head. "Kansas and, indeed, the nation are watching our progress," Reed observed. "We must not fail because of personal prejudice, parochialism, or sectional rivalry."[163]

One sectional rivalry that did remain was that between KU and WSU. The impression by some in the community was that the exact relationship between KU and WSU was not clear "and not well understood by either university."[164] Certainly, there were some gray areas, and some watching and waiting to see how things evolved with the various constituencies. And those constituencies were divided. Some Wichita physicians, for example, were uncertain about the WSU connection, feeling that if a full-fledged medical school with a full teaching hospital facility were impractical in Wichita, it was best to stick with a pure KU connection. And the interinstitutional personal dynamics changed as the administration at KU changed.

Part of the pressure concerned facilities. Dr. George Platt, who had come with Ahlberg from Syracuse, recognized that one difficulty with a joint venture concerned physical facilities. No one thought the houses were adequate, and WSU was slow, partly because funding from the legislature was not forthcoming, to come up with a suitable alternative on campus. Some local physicians, meanwhile, were not sure that a building at WSU, particularly in the interior of the campus where access for patients for a clinic might be difficult and proximity to hospitals marginal, would be the solution.[165]

It was never certain with all concerned that the physical location of KUSM-W would continue to be on the WSU campus. There was a good deal of public talk that it would be, as in the Reed interview, but there is ample evidence that KUMC and the state legislature had as an early priority the purchase or construction of the "neutral" facility, independent of WSU, that Rieke had mentioned in his first "understandings" with Reed.

The old Sedgwick County Hospital, which had just been renamed E.B. Allen Hospital after an early local physician, was the choice. It had been tax supported by the county since the 1920s, the current structure at Ninth and Minneapolis Streets having been completed in 1953. It had been 61,000 square feet originally, but a 14,000-plus square foot annex had been added later. By the 1970s there were 150 beds there. While it was becoming more and more run down, the Board of Regents architects found it to be structurally sound.[166] There was good space for conversion and it was fairly convenient to the major hospitals, though not much more convenient than WSU being in basically the same northeast quadrant of town as the university, albeit somewhat further south in the direction of Wesley, the VA, and St. Joseph, and somewhat further west in the direction of St. Francis.[167]

In the fall of 1972, a group that included Ahlberg, Reed, and Rieke, met with a committee from the state legislature headed by Wichitan Roger Turner. Its agenda was to prepare a proposal for the Kansas Board of Regents that the state purchase the county hospital and modify it to serve as offices and classrooms for KUSM-W. The hospital had been running a $50,000 a month deficit caring for fewer than 100 chronically ill patients, and it seemed that such a change would be beneficial to all.[168] Turner's committee proposed that the local mill levy supporting the hospital be left in place until 1978 as a means of aiding in the transition, and that some county medical services could remain for a time until KUSM-W grew into the space.[169]

There were some problems. The condition of E.B. Allen Hospital was poor. It was an all-electric facility, something that did not bode well for operating costs in the middle of the 1973 energy crisis. The county could not afford to install the diesel generators needed for back-up electric

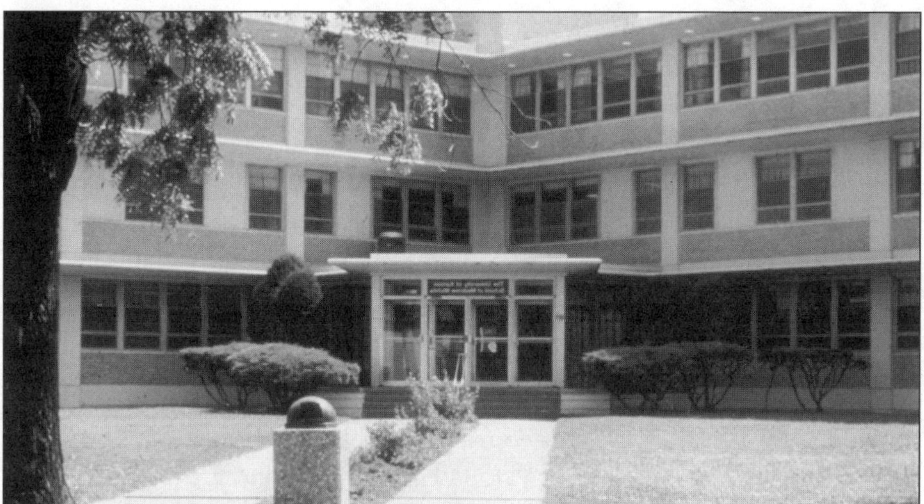

E.B. Allen Hospital

power.[170] E.B. Allen was not then well adapted to use by the medical school, and it was not certain how well a transition period would work, with the county still housing patients there. And there were legal difficulties. One was that the land had originally come from an estate, and the transfer had specified that it was to be used by the county strictly for medical purposes. Would a slight change in use cause the land to revert to the original owners? Also it appeared that the sale or transfer of property valued at more than $20,000 by the county would require a countywide election. Third, the probate court of Sedgwick County had a legal obligation to treat alcoholics and mental patients. Should E.B. Allen be entirely converted to an institution of higher education, where would this be done?[171]

Reed said that the medical school could offer this service indefinitely.[172] But Rieke was concerned about having patients at the Wichita school. That was certainly not in the original "community-based" mission as it had been sold to the hospitals, and he feared that "some of its implications will just destroy our relationship" with those hospitals. The universities involved, Rieke said in February 1973, do not want "a state subsidized hospital in competition with our friends there." He also did not like references in the press, and in legislation introduced by the Sedgwick County delegation in Topeka, to the "Wichita State University Medical Center." That language implied a full-range hospital and minimized KU's role.[173]

Turner introduced a bill in the legislature early in 1973 providing for the transfer of E.B. Allen Hospital to the state.[174] However, at that point the initiative failed when it died in the House Ways and Means Committee. The official explanation was that WSU had not provided the required feasibility study. But word was that there were significant roadblocks, poor communication, and not much enthusiasm. It would be over a year before the matter could be taken up again.[175] A feasibility report on E.B. Allen did reach the Board of Regents in November 1973. It set remodeling costs at $604,000 and operating costs at $558,000 a year. There would remain a thirty-five bed, long-term care unit, a twenty bed alcoholic holding unit, and a thirty-two bed mental holding unit. It did not seem an auspicious scenario.[176]

These negotiations about an off-campus site did not imply that WSU was to have no connection. WSU was still in the name and WSU officials were directly involved in the planning for a possible move to E.B. Allen. When the immediate plan for transfer collapsed with faculty coming on board and student arrival postponed from summer 1973 to January 1974, WSU provided a stopgap facility where KUSM-W could at least get started as an operating entity. Fairmount Towers was a privately owned dormitory across Hillside Avenue from WSU to the west. In the spring of 1973, an arrangement was made for KUSM-W to move its headquarters to the fifth floor of that facility.[177] Meanwhile the $4.4 million Life Science Building at WSU, which had been discussed as a future home for KUSM-W, was nearing completion.[178]

Fairmount Towers was no more an ideal home than was E.B. Allen in its current state. If, as C. Northcutt Parkinson says, a perfect headquarters is a sign of a decaying organization, KUSM-W, at this time must have been healthy indeed. The growing staff adapted and did not complain, but co-existing with a college dormitory was not what anyone had in mind. Many remembered the sound of guitars, the smell of marijuana, and the concern about security associated with that dormitory environment.[179] Dr. Richard Guthrie thought it not "too conducive," as on Monday morning he had to make his way to his office by way of "elevators full of discarded refuse and chicken bones."[180]

First the school had half the fifth floor, then all of it, and shortly expanded to the whole third floor as well. They configured it as best they could with a small library/conference room, while looking for something better. Jerry Lessard, who had a master's in education, was the first full-time professional employee of the school hired, as he remembered, by a man with a "distinctive voice," who met him in the living room of a small house with papers piled all about. Lessard remembered the dorm as "exciting." The KUSM-W staff was coming to work while the students were going out to school, and there were many questions about the presence of all those adults.

Reed set the tone for the rest by seeming perfectly comfortable with what he called this "plain pipe rack" surrounding. It did not need to be fancy, he said, as they were given there the opportunity to do exciting work.[181] RoxAnn Dicker, who worked with the outreach program, remembered that there were file cabinets in bathtubs next to each office at Fairmount Towers but that Reed was convinced it was "ideal office space." What made it ideal, no doubt, was the "air of expectation and electricity" that Dicker remembered as being even stronger than the odors. There were meetings in the hallways and parking lots. Reed and his wife Geney would have barbecues and casserole gatherings for the staff at their home, and "we would talk and dream in the back yard."[182]

That the physical offices of KUSM-W remained on the WSU campus did not, however, mean that those in Kansas City accepted a strong and continuing WSU role in the operation. In August 1973, for example, Ahlberg wrote a memo that the press said "was interpreted by some officials as the first step to try to convert the Wichita branch of the KU Medical School into the WSU School of Medicine." This involved appointing Reed to the new WSU post of Vice President for Health Education, while appointing Carmen Ness to take his old job of dean of WSU's CHRP. Ahlberg proposed at that point that KU should appoint a new dean for KUSM-W who would report to Reed along with the CHRP dean. "Placing the head of a part of the KU Medical School under a WSU vice president," the *Lawrence Daily Journal* crowed, "in the proposed way, led some involved with the situation to conclude WSU would be over a major hurdle and, at the least, well on its way toward what it has long desired: Its own medical school." Sources said that Ahlberg had not informed KU Chancellor Dykes before making his proposal public.

Dykes responded that whoever might be dean at KUSM-W would report to the vice chancellor at KUMC as usual and not to any WSU official, even if it were Reed. Ahlberg countered that it was fine for Reed to remain in his dean's position and report to Rieke in Kansas City at least until 1975, but at that point Ahlberg wanted Reed to devote his full time to WSU health education programs. "Ahlberg's administrative proposal," wrote the press, "reliable sources say, was further evidence of WSU's intention to become as full-fledged a university as KU." Ahlberg had asked the Regents to delay approval of expansion of the KU law school until the feasibility of a WSU law school could be studied. He, however, denied to reporters that WSU was trying to control the clinical branch in Wichita or that he and the university were in any way in league with the Wichita Chamber of Commerce. The Lawrence reporter, however, concluded that "the Wichita school is striking out on an independent course to build its offering irrespective of coordinated statewide academic planning initiated by the regents." And he averred that there was strong community support for this in the Air Capital.[183] Reed did become Vice President for Health Education at Wichita, but he remained also dean of KUSM-W.[184]

Some of the faculty at Kansas City responded to these aspersions with a sneer. Dr. Robert Manning recalled that there was fear of siphoning money from the Kansas City campus and concern about "the academic level that could be attained and maintained in Wichita."[185] Dr. Joseph Meek noticed the same atmosphere. The stationery with the WSU name on it "really frosted" people in Kansas City, as did the location at Fairmount Hall and the planning for a new building for KUSM-W on the WSU campus. Meanwhile, "paranoia was so rampant" in Wichita that people there took every fear about scarce funding and duplication as a personal slam on their ambitions and good offices for the state. Meek observed that other schools in the state feared Wichita also. Fort Hays State University, for instance, wanted the nurses training part of the money package and did not want WSU to have "anything that looked or smelled like a medical school." KU was "looking down its nose" at family practice, while Wichita recognized that "there was political hay to be made from espousing that viewpoint." It was Meek's opinion that institutional enmity was strong enough that if the fate of KUSM-W had been left to WSU and KU "they would probably have made a flop of it," but the community of doctors and hospitals in Wichita and elsewhere wanted it to survive and so did the state government. KU and WSU "would probably be fighting to this day otherwise."[186]

The immediate task for Reed, in light of all this, was to collect a faculty with not only legitimacy, but credibility as academics as well as practitioners. The department chairs would be particularly key elements in this, though Reed did not have the money or the "perks" to attract a complete range of full-time people to these positions. He and the chairs then had to create a curriculum that balanced the unique elements in Wichita's mission with traditional medical school requirements. Here he had to balance the criticisms of some in Kansas City, that Wichita would be second-rate academically with no research presence and only a mentorship program where the students would follow physicians on grand rounds. The critics in the legislature meanwhile were pushing for a curriculum that was almost pure application. Reed had to defend with this latter group the idea that KUSM-W could not meet accreditation requirements with a pure emphasis on family practice, but must take students through clinical rotations in fields such as surgery, pediatrics, internal medicine, and obstetrics and gynecology. For his determination that they needed some additional training to be complete human beings and good citizens he had no particular political constituency, only his strong personal conviction. But he was determined to accomplish that also.

What emerged was impressive to almost everyone who evaluated it. Every chair was a unique negotiation and a customized package.

Dr. Gayle Stephens was an obvious choice to head the Department of Family Practice. He was the first faculty appointed by Reed, in July of 1972, and actually reported to the little house on the campus, moving to Huntsville in June of 1973 just as the move to Fairmount Towers was made. He taught some classes in CHRP, met with local physicians, and worked on the curriculum. Stephens, definitely a Wichita partisan, thought KU had usurped a WSU initiative, but remembered that Reed then, as was true of him later, played the politics of it close to the vest and kept the faculty out of any institutional or administrative squabbles. Reed, Stephens said, "interpreted everything that happened in Kansas City," and interpreted it in the positive and enthusiastic way characteristic of a builder.[187] The successor to Dr. Stephens as the family practice chair was Dr. Billy Gardner.[188]

The arrangement with Stephens was fairly typical of these early negotiations. He was to be paid $35,000 the first year, which was more than Reed was making, and was to be permitted to earn up to $4,000 a year in clinical activity. He would have WSU benefits and group insurance rates, and would have a joint appointment at CHRP, where he might also teach. "As previously discussed," Reed added, "because of the unique character of your participation in the WSU branch, and because your acceptance of this appointment is contingent on several factors over which neither of us control, I propose that we review the terms of this agreement at the end of the first year of our association." Reed could not give Stephens a job description. He pointed out that until the students arrived he would have many and varied responsibilities.[189]

Faculty recruitment in general was a challenge. Reed wrote Dr. Daniel Roberts, who was in charge of the faculty reimbursement committee, that the problems of faculty reimbursement were so "formidable" that "any reasonable pin pointing of responsibility appears impossible." Roberts's committee could not be expected to "address in a meaningful way" the long-range problems of faculty reimbursement in Wichita. However, unless some understanding could be reached with the hospitals to accept KUSM-W faculty into hospital clinic and outpatient areas to provide agreed upon fee services "there is little reason for inviting prospective faculty for interviews."[190] Direct state compensation would not be adequate. Reed contacted the Medical Society of Sedgwick County about volunteer faculty. He reminded them that, in November 1971, about 60 percent of Medical Society members had expressed an interest in volunteering. However, "it is not possible to set forth in a memorandum . . . all the provisions governing the awarding of academic titles, the basis for part-time paid appointments, etc." All he could do was send out a questionnaire asking local physicians to reaffirm their interest in "a teaching-learning experience not directly related to one of the major teaching disciplines," and to say how many hours they could devote to didactic lectures, scheduled ward rounds and conferences or student advising.[191] Within a year, it became policy that people contributing fewer than fifty hours a year (and there were 200 of these in 1974) would not be reimbursed and would have the uniform title of clinical associate.[192] The school also set a standard base for full-time, twelve-month work at $25,000, and part-time at some percentage of that.[193] Otherwise every step would have to be custom made.

Dr. Richard Guthrie was the first chair of the Department of Pediatrics. He came from Missouri for an interview in November 1972 and was offered the job in December. He did not accept at first, but after consideration did accept in January 1973. Guthrie had a contract with the University of Missouri running until September 1, so until that time he commuted to Wichita and to the house on 17th Street. His first office when he settled in Wichita was in Fairmount Towers.

Guthrie was different than some in that he had an academic background, never having been in private practice, and he was a full-time faculty member. Although one might not guess it to meet him in the twenty-first century, Guthrie claims that he was rather shy at that period. He had never had an administrative position and found going out to meet the public and potential faculty members daunting. He did meet all the pediatricians in town, asking them what role they would like to have

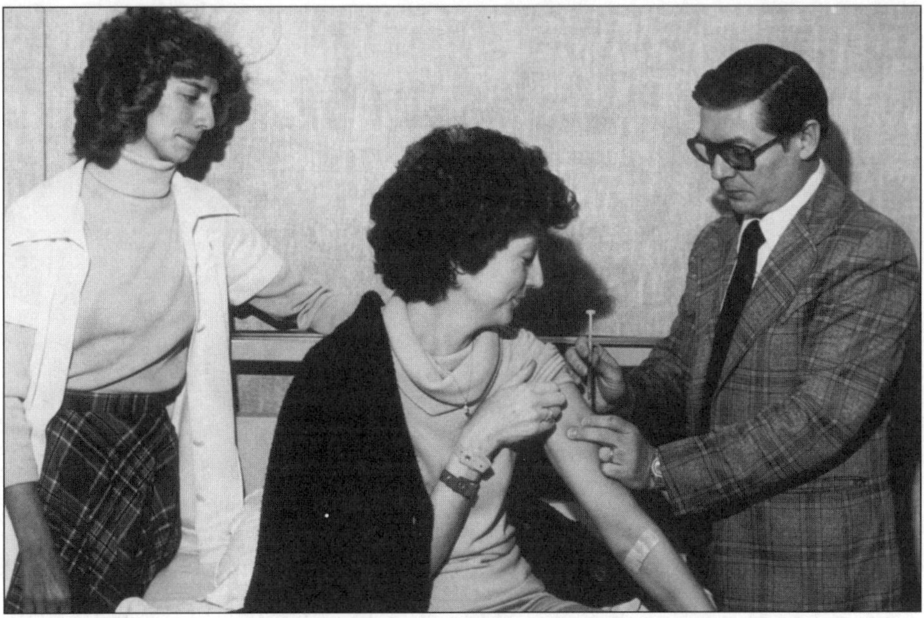

In 1980, Richard Guthrie, M.D., administered the world's first injection of biosynthetic human insulin.

and what type of faculty they would like him to recruit. He also asked them and community members what was needed in the community in the way of enhancements to the pediatric specialty. Guthrie developed into a "forceful personality," to use his own words, but just one among several represented by the early department chairs. "This was an experiment," he said, but "we had to be forceful personalities to make this work."

It became a personal experiment for Guthrie as well. He became interested in the self-treatment of diabetes, developed a large patient base in that area while at KUSM-W, and eventually moved into full-time private practice outside his original specialty and in a way that he did not expect at all when he accepted the academic position at Wichita in 1973.[194]

Dr. Ernest Crow became chair of the Department of Internal Medicine, quite reluctantly. Dr. David Robinson, who by then had replaced Rieke at KUMC, called Crow and spoke to him persuasively about being department chair. Crow agreed, then overnight thought better of it and called Reed the next day. Reed made him chair of the search committee, but it turned out that the person whom they hired, Dr. Arnold Greenhouse, stayed only a few days. With plans far along, Crow stepped into the gap until someone else could be found. Crow felt that he did not have the proper academic background for the job and that academic and research credentials would be important, especially in the field of internal medicine, for gaining peer status with Kansas City faculty. He also had an active local practice with a specialty in cardiology, which he was loathe to abandon.

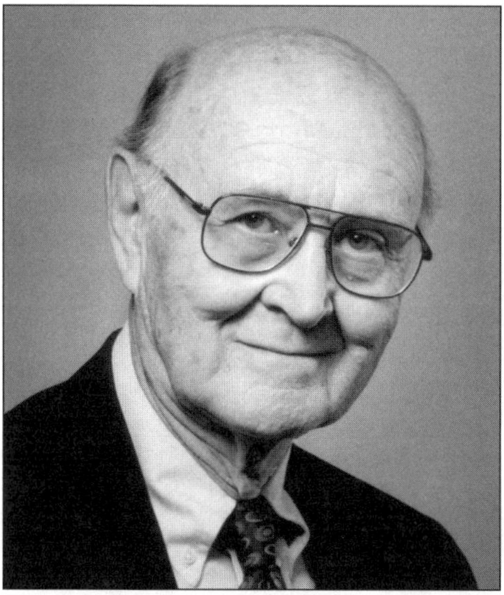

Ernest Crow, M.D.

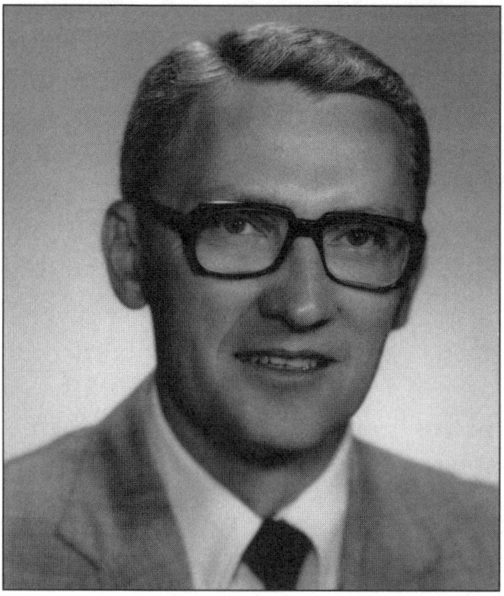

Douglas Voth, M.D.

Crow remained one year, aided by Dr. Alan Forker in a part-time role, before he was replaced in the fall of 1974 by Dr. Douglas Voth, who had been a leading candidate in the original search, but who did not accept the post at that time. Voth, like Guthrie, was full-time and had a strong academic background, so these two had a special bond. Crow formed a number of committees, the members of which sat down with a textbook in internal medicine and worked out a curriculum. The Department of Internal Medicine was truly citywide, with students rotating through all the hospitals, so Crow from his office in Fairmount Towers did a lot of coordination and developed a lot of urban public relations. He was a local man, a known and respected quantity, something that was important to getting the program up and going. Curriculum development and faculty recruiting, as with all departments, was essential and pioneering work.[195]

The two other department heads hired initially (all four chairs were on board by February 1973) were in surgery and obstetrics and gynecology.[196] In both cases the department heads were giants in influence in the Wichita medical community as well as men of charismatic personality, prosperous private practices, and strong personal opinion and direction. Dr. George Farha took the chairmanship of the Department of Surgery and Dr. Daniel Roberts the Department of Obstetrics and Gynecology. Both had academic credentials and publications. Farha had thirty or forty papers on general surgery—"nothing earthshaking," he would say, "but a little bit stimulating." He also had a most successful surgery practice, at one time the largest purely surgical group in the U.S., run with his brother Jim. Roberts was not only board certified in two specialties (obstetrics and gynecology and pathology), but had a Ph.D. in anatomy, was an expert in electron microscopy, was a great writer of successful grants, and had a considerable background and achievement in research. However, the most notable characteristic of both was their success as clinicians, as fundraisers and moneymakers, and as recognizers and recruiters of talent. There were debates about whether these men could have tenure at KU since they were only part-time employees. Neither much

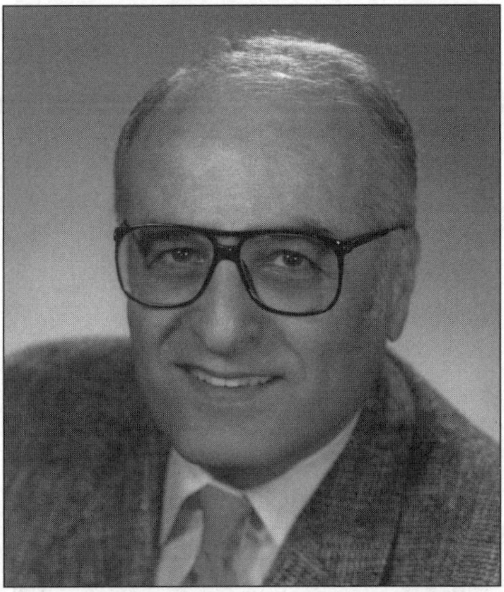

George Farha, M.D.

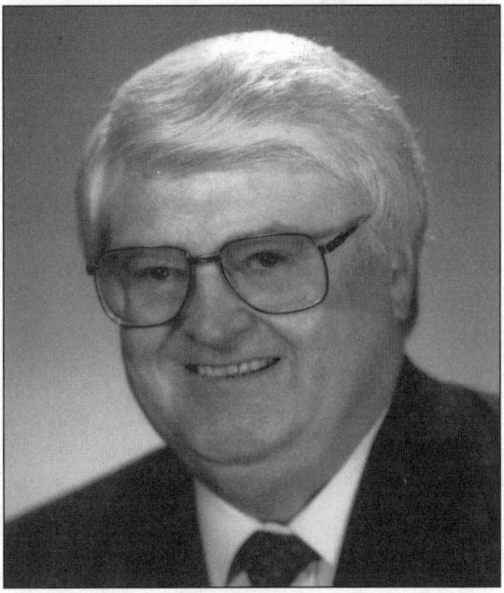

Daniel Roberts, M.D.

cared. They both emphasized that medicine was a continuum and that the strict divisions in the mind of some between clinical practice and the academic side were artificial. They were most dedicated to the idea of having an educational component in Wichita but thought the fertilization would run both ways. "Don't judge us by titles, but by performance," Farha said. If the new professors and department chairs did not do the job, he said, no one would have to fire them. They would resign.[197] Dr. Robert Manning recalled that, to put it mildly, these men were not "subservient personalities," and had no interest in developing subservient programs. "If you wanted something done you got Roberts and Farha on your side and you had a chance of getting it done."[198]

Roberts was particularly meteoric—a "whirling dervish at times," Dr. Robert Manning recalled—and also a "consummate politician." Roy House, the chief administrator at Wesley and the man who brought Roberts to Wichita, said it was his job to put Roberts's many talents to work and to "hold him down in some areas and let him go in others."[199] Reed had a similar task. When Roberts died while still in his fifties in 1994, his memorial booklet contained the slogan, "*Dum Spiro Spero*—While I breathe, I hope."[200] A man driven, Roberts once told a reporter, "I want to accomplish everything. I enjoy, I just enjoy making things happen." Dr. Reed described Roberts as "a very aggressive person injected into a very comfortable community."[201] Roberts's wife recalled that "nobody wanted to take him on," but remembered too "how great a time that was" when Farha and Roberts joined the team at KUSM-W. They were sometimes silently referred to as the "Lebanese and Irish godfathers." Certainly both were most self-assured, "benevolent dictators" with lots of down-to-earth experience. They were determined that Wichita not be treated "like sort of a poor stepchild" by the residents of any ivory tower, and they had the credentials to go with their *chutzpah*. They suggested that any students who might come to Wichita with a negative attitude could just "check their attitude and their sandals and white socks at the door" and get with the program. That not enough KU students would choose to come was a possibility this cadre of zealots never seriously considered.[202]

Dr. Dean Schwartz, who served on the faculty search advisory committee for KUSM-W in 1972, affirmed that every practicing physician he talked to "considered it part of his mission to teach." The response of the medical community in Wichita, not only to opportunities to serve on the faculty part-time but to serve as volunteers, was overwhelmingly positive. Schwartz got the impression that "KC was looking down their nose at Wichita. They did not have a lot of hope for a branch down here." But the combination of the great "clinical possibilities," the fine faculty cadre, and the enthusiastic participation made him think the prospects were strong.[203]

Indeed, things had moved. Rieke wrote to Wes Sowers and others in the state legislature in January 1973, emphasizing that while the funding for KUSM-W might be well hidden in Governor Docking's budget, it was very much there. "It is a coordinated, cohesive master plan which is well along in its implementation and should not be viewed as benefiting one geographic area of the state more than another." Cooperation between Wichita and Lawrence and Kansas City was, Rieke said, "very good, indeed," and funds allocated on paper to KUMC were flowing in large amounts to Wichita and other Kansas cities. For example in fiscal year 1972, more than $171,000 was paid by KUMC to three Wichita hospitals for house staff stipends, and $45,000 more went to support faculty in Wichita. During fiscal year 1973, $285,000 was allocated for house staff support at Wichita, and $265,000 for faculty and operating expense. Rieke noted that Reed could not recruit enough faculty to fully use the financial support in that category. "It should be emphasized that even though faculty in our branch in Wichita number less than 1 percent of our faculty in Kansas City, nearly 5 percent of KUMC's total state appropriation is targeted for Wichita this year." The next year would be more significant still, with more than $750,000 allocated to Wichita.[204]

Dr. George Dyck became chairman of the Department of Psychiatry in June of 1973, just as the move to Fairmount Towers was taking place. Dyck had been working at the Prairie View mental health facility in Newton. He contacted Dr. Reed because he was looking for new challenges, but had not thought of working at KUSM-W full time, much less heading a new department. But he found that Reed was "the kind of person who motivates you to do a good job." After an initial period of feeling inadequate to the task, partly because he felt he had less academic background than some of the others, Dyck got into the swing of things with the support of the rest of the team. "You have to establish your own territory in order to have the ability to accomplish things," he remembered later of those times.[205]

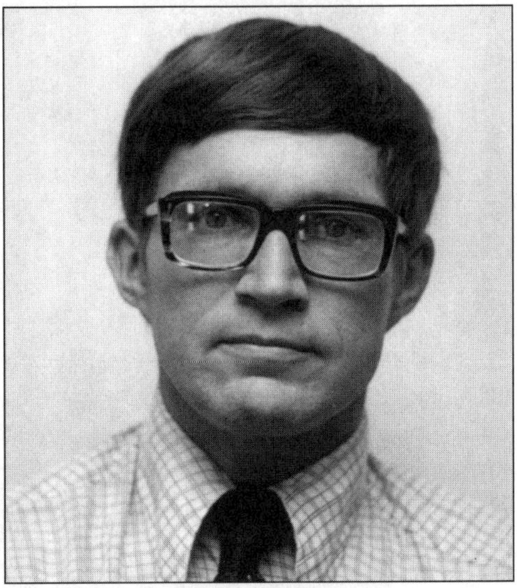

George Dyck, M.D.

With pediatrics and psychiatry, the new departments were establishing residencies for the first time in Wichita rather than being able to depend on existing graduate programs, as was the case with other departments. That, of course, was one of the advantages hospitals and the profession locally saw in the establishment of the school in the first place. There was a strong correlation between the location where residents took their training and where they eventually practiced.

That same spring of 1973, when Dyck was appointed, came three other key employees who were to exercise some considerable influence. Dr. Joseph Dominic had been a member of the faculty of the Department of English at WSU and became the director of student services and program development at KUSM-W. Lorene Valentine, formerly with the WSU CHRP office, took over accounting and business affairs.[206] Dr. Dean Kortge, a Ph.D. in history, became Director of Special Projects with responsibility for publicity and outreach. Jerry Lessard, who also came from a non-medical background and from WSU, worked closely with this group, as did Vince Marshall, hired in July 1974 to develop the educational technology aspect of the school.[207] Lessard remembered that they were all "young Turks" who were interested in the "human dimensions in medical education" and as a consequence "raised some eyebrows" among physicians in town.[208]

They were all non-traditional in a way. Clearly two doctoral degrees in the humanities and a master's in education were not the type that usually came to the top of the hiring list at medical schools. Only Valentine seemed to fit a traditional hiring slot, but it was not exactly

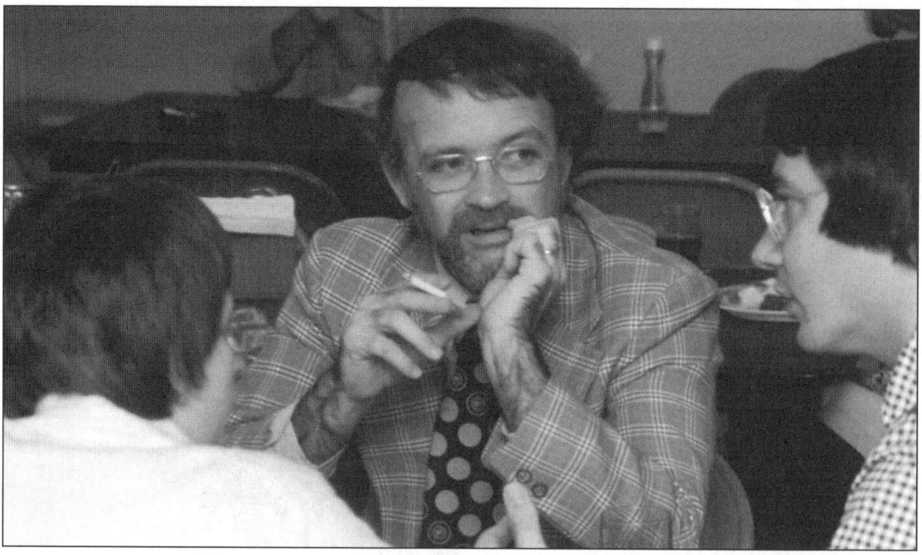

Dean Kortge, Ph.D.

standard practice at the time to assign a young woman, not far out of college, such significant financial responsibilities. In all these cases, it was a matter of Reed's ability to judge the person independently of hard and fast rules or precedents. And he demanded enthusiasm and energy. RoxAnn Dicker remembered that Reed "did not hire anyone who just wanted a job."[209] All of these staff employees were in their twenties.

Kortge was painting houses at the time, fell off a ladder and broke his wrist, and needed the money. Reed was interested in a hypertension screening project and had received funding to use a recreational vehicle (it turned out to be a Winnebago) to test thousands of Kansans where

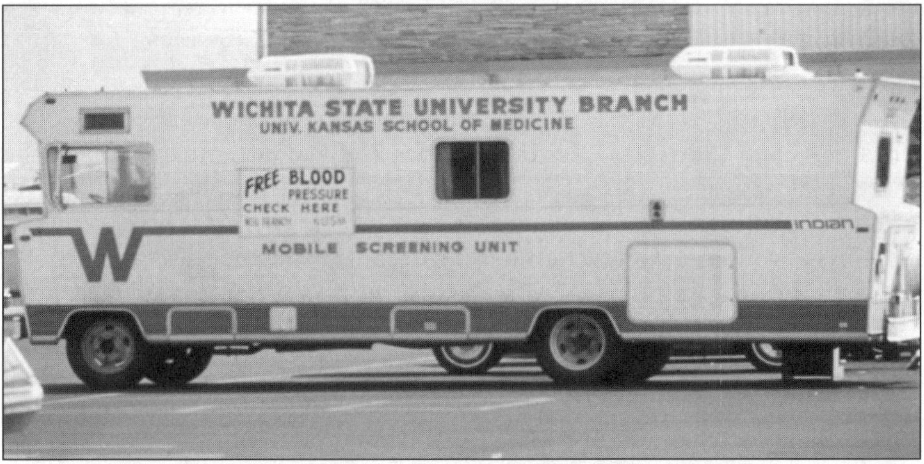

The Winnebago used for an outreach hypertension screening project.

they lived. Kortge not only convinced Reed that he would work cheaper than an M.D. and do just as well but that he understood and could sell Reed's concept of outreach. Reed wanted medical students to "get the sense of being in a real community, breaking away from the mold of being in a medical school only." Kortge worked with preceptorships, where students could interact with physicians in rural areas, networking with the CHRP program so that those people and the medical students could be "in a practice setting where they could rub shoulders with one another and break down barriers." He helped organize fairs and dinners to break down barriers between doctors, students, and community leaders. He organized workshops in Dodge City, Harper, Kingman, Pratt, and other western Kansas cities using KUSM-W faculty. He eventually screened about 250,000 people with the van. He remembered it was "kind of like a circus," but that it was also fun and useful. Reed was not sure what Kortge's role would be exactly ("we did some pretty crazy things") but he was willing to trust the person and to let it develop in an entrepreneurial way. "Go forth and do no evil," he told his new recycled historian.[210]

Joe Dominic had a special interest in what motivates people to become powerful learners, and he was attracted by the opportunity to create an environment in which motivated people could learn more than they might have imagined possible. Among other things that came out of this thinking was something called Interphase, a break between clinical rotations in which the medical students at Wichita would be exposed to humanistic issues such as their personal reaction to death. It was important, Dominic thought, that the new doctors not be simply "overwhelmed by the scientific part." In this he had the support of Reed, who himself had a talent, Dominic remembered, to get people to "own the values he had." Things happened at Wichita as a result of a certain style, and Reed set that tone and style from the start.[211]

Valentine had been a secretary with KUMC on some grant-funded projects as early as 1969, and rose in the world by her merits. She knew physicians and they respected her abilities and she became eventually the first female associate dean for KUSM-W.[212] When she left KUSM-W in 1982, Valentine became chief operating officer (COO) of Health Frontiers, a multi-hospital purchasing organization. She was then COO of St. Francis Health Corporation before returning to KUSM-W as head of Rural Health Education and Services in 1990. Her career illustrates that Reed was a good judge of potential. All of his cadre of young employees have continued in responsible positions since those days, and most have risen very far indeed.

Certainly the new faculty got out in the community along with Reed to promote and explain the school. Reed spoke to the West Side Lions in April 1972 on "The Unique Role of the Wichita State University Branch of the University of Kansas School of Medicine."[213] The next month he did a workshop on "The Community, a Base for Undergraduate Medical Education," sponsored by the College of Human Medicine at Michigan State University. He was appointed to develop and implement for the Association of Schools of Allied Health Professions and the Bureau of Health Manpower Education of the National Institutes of Health a series of two-and-a-half day programs to be conducted on campuses across the nation in 1972 and 1973.[214] The Department of Health Education and Welfare appointed him to the National Advisory Allied Health Related Professions Council of the National Institutes of Health.[215] He spoke in the fall of 1972 to the combined medical societies of southeast Kansas on "The Role of the Community Hospital in Medical and Allied Health Education," and to the Kansas Chapter of the American College of Surgeons on "The Role of the WSU Branch of KUSM in Undergraduate and Graduate Medical Education."[216] Dr. Stephens spoke to the North Wichita Kiwanis Club in September 1972 on "Development of the WSU

Medical Branch."[217] In October, he was in Garden City appearing before the medical staff of St. Catherine's Hospital speaking about developments in family practice education at the WSU Branch and discussing "possible cooperative efforts between the branch and the Garden City medical community."[218] This activity continued to be frequent in 1973. Reed spoke to the AMA annual Congress of Medical Education in Chicago in February on "Integrated Teaching in Medicine and Allied Health," and to the Wichita Downtown Lions on "Medical Education at WSU-Where Do We Stand?" Stephens spoke to WSU's Phil Delta Kappa Chapter on "Development of the WSU Branch Medical School."[219] These are only some of the examples of a continuing public relations presence in town and around the nation.

The content of at least one of these speeches, the one before the AMA in Chicago, survives. Reed spoke there about the "territoriality" that had characterized medicine, to its detriment in his view. Specialists tended to exclude general practitioners, dental hygienists warred with dental assistants, as did medical technologists with medical laboratory technicians. "Professional nursing groups are convinced that the physician looks upon a nurse as his personal servant and not as a colleague and equal." In general, Reed said, there was too much "professional over protection," and this was a deterrent "to the establishment of a logical system of providing quality health care." Too often there were eleven quarterbacks and no blockers. The whole profession was producer rather than consumer-oriented and there was "timidity" about changing that through pragmatism and innovation. Medical students needed to get off campuses. Most of them had been "educated in academic isolation," a practice "difficult to defend." The medical school admission system, Reed thought, tended to reward the best scientist "over another with less elegant science background, but with more demonstrable humanistic attributes and interests." This led to the mistaken idea that medicine was self-sufficient. "Demonstrable evidence and academic achievement must become his way of life—there is little time for introspection and establishment of meaningful interpersonal relations with professional peers—in short, he becomes a 'loner.'" Many were unprepared for the emotional upheavals encountered in medical school—the first human anatomical dissection, the first clinical assignment to a child with an incurable disease, the first encounter with violent death. Without specific attention to these, the student might develop a façade of pseudo-superiority and self-sufficiency rather than warmth and understanding. In other words medical school could be dehumanizing. Reed quoted Dr. Leonard Finninger, who said, "The aim of education is the development of the capacity to learn so that one may adapt to change with judgment and vision." Health care teams should learn to work together as students so they could work together later. And surely humanistic skills were directly and obviously useful in an atmosphere of high malpractice liability.[220] Such a speech as this was a good summary of some of Reed's goals for KUSM-W and a good guide to the type of influence his personality and philosophy had on the developing institutional culture there.

In the summer of 1973, a policy was drafted for compensation of certain members of the faculty doing limited practice at the branch facility. Establishing practices to supplement the budget was a standard feature in traditional medical school teaching hospitals, but KUSM-W's mission as a "community-based" school made the matter of potential competition with private hospitals a delicate one. Reed wrote Rieke: "Adequate and proper compensation for members of the clinical faculty at the University of Kansas School of Medicine-Wichita State University Branch is a difficult and complicated matter." There was a "marked disproportion" between the level of salaries the state could provide to highly trained and educated faculty members and the income that any competent physician could make. The "geographical full-time" system introduced at KUMC in 1948 seemed to have worked well, and allowing some practice would help supplement the $25,000 salary approved for full-time faculty at Wichita. Geographical full-time would allow people who were paid part-time salaries by the university to engage in private practice in conjunction with and supplemental to their teaching. These faculty members would be limited in the time they could spend thus, and the income they could make, and their patients could be available for the teaching functions of the branch. Overhead would be paid and salaries supplemented by the WSU Branch accounting office and the WSU Endowment Association in the short term and probably by a professional association or corporation in the long run.[221] These arrangements did not apply to the true part-time faculty who had special contracts and already established independent practices, which they were allowed to continue. There would be growing pains, wrote Dr. Thomas Hurst, president of the Medical Society of Sedgwick County, but "having a medical school could improve the stature, quality, and character of medicine in the area."[222]

Reed wrote his friend Dr. Robert Evans in Rockford in October 1973 that he was struggling to smooth out several bumps in the road. Hospitals in Wichita had a long tradition of graduate medical education "and until very recently they have presumed that this should continue to be their prerogative" and that maybe KUSM-W should deal only with undergraduates. "Of course they have no objection to accepting the full $9,500 per position that the state is making available; they simply don't believe we should exercise any control over their programs." Liability insurance for students was presenting a problem. Wichita had high malpractice exposure "because of some very active plaintive-type attorneys" who had obtained large judgments against local hospitals. Most local doctors supported the program, but some felt they should be reimbursed for even hourly contact with students, something the budget did not allow. It would be, Reed thought, "a very expensive proposition."[223]

Evans reassured him on some of these points. Perhaps part of the problem was the "branch" designation, which Reed might have "to fight with great vigor since it provides a formal support for a very basic fear which many practitioner-teachers will continue to have until the school has been shown to be innocuous many years in the future." The graduate education issue would resolve itself, as the trend in the country was toward connection of these programs with universities and not just with hospitals. "The simple truth is that they need your *imprimatur* to continue to exist." The expense would not be so great. Wichita would not have research and other facilities costs and undergraduate education was far less expensive than graduate. "I have the feeling that the physicians at Wichita are trying to extract from you a series of ironclad promises which you cannot give. I think they need to be told this and be told that it is their involvement, which guarantees the answers to their questions and not your simple promise. This has to be said hundreds of times and become a litany which they eventually accept."[224]

Curriculum included the traditional topics and more. Reed early in 1973 talked to the press about possible courses in human sexuality, human growth and development, drug abuse, and ecology, as well as mobile clinics for continuing education of physicians and nurses and primary education of the public. Then there was the Interphase idea. The curriculum at KUSM-W, he emphasized, did not have to be the same as in Kansas City, but just "equivalent."[225]

The student body started to form. Wichita had, in the summer of 1973, a list of thirty-eight students from the Kansas City campus who expressed an interest in filling one of the sixteen slots available for the first class at KUSM-W. Most explained their interest by stating that they wanted to see how medicine was practiced outside a university-based medical center, as they felt that was more likely to parallel their own eventual practices.[226] By fall, plans were firm for the first class, which was to start in January 1974. They would spend six to ten weeks in a clerkship in each specialty at the four hospitals in town that were participating. There would be forty electives in such specialties as radiology and plastic surgery. During the first twelve months of the eighteen-month program each student would spend one-half day a week in a community physician's office getting experience with ambulatory care patients. Over 150 doctors were participating in this. During the final four weeks there would be preceptorships in doctors' offices, primarily in rural areas. The Interphase between the clerkships would emphasize the psychological and social aspects of health care. Reed could not tell the press at this point where the future home of his school would be. The feasibility of both E.B. Allen and a building on campus were still under investigation.[227] Wherever it was, the unique features of KUSM-W were that it would be "community-based," and "practice-oriented," with an emphasis on the primary care role of the physician. "Basically," Reed said, "we are not trying to make medical experts out of our students, although the program is designed in such a way that any graduate can specialize if that is what he is interested in."[228]

As the students arrived and began their program in the early months of 1974, controversy still swirled around KUSM-W in several areas. Some legislators were concerned about perceived abuses with the KUMC Physician Practice Corporation, where the average salary in 1974 was $34,000 with the state paying only about $8,000 of that. Some called for more audits and control of practice income, however advantageous that might be to the support of the school. However, that was difficult, given the part-time arrangements of many faculty in Wichita who had genuinely independent practices.[229]

Then there was a furor on the question of how much emphasis there should be in Wichita on family practice. The rural press continued to be concerned that, during the past twenty years, 64 percent of the medical school graduates had left the state and few who stayed were in primary care or serving in rural areas. "Public needs," said one paper, "play second fiddle." The state needed "more doctors who treat mumps, measles and bellyache, who bind our wounds, deliver our babies, monitor our heart attacks, prescribe our medicines, and practice preventative medicine to keep us well in the first place."[230] Dr. Victor Vorhees told a reporter, "We have an opportunity in Wichita to develop a new kind of medical center. Unfortunately, WSU is requiring students to take all specialties except family practice." Dr. Stephens agreed, "The way I see the branch developing is in a very traditional imitation of the University of Kansas Medical Center. . . . The State of Kansas cannot justify spending the amount of money and effort it will spend in Wichita to increase the number of medical school graduates by thirty or fifty or so a year if they produce the same choice of doctors who are going to live in the same places. The state is not going to be better off." Dr. Dominic replied that both KUMC and KUSM-W had tried to develop programs to expose students to rural practice. Wesley itself offered residencies in family practice in Phillipsburg, Belleville, Coffeyville, and Minneola, and it was imagined that this program would be fully integrated with the KUSM-W system. Reed responded that family practice still lacked credibility and that "it would be suicide for a new school to be designated a family practice school." Only eight of the 114 medical schools in the nation required any study of family practice. KUSM-W was trying to make its family practice clerkship attractive enough that students would want to take it.[231] "Because we live in a democracy," Reed pointed out, "we can't just assign a doctor to a place—we don't assign plumbers."[232]

There was still the KU/WSU/KUSM-W administrative issue. "In moments of despair," Reed wrote, "it has seemed that our most productive efforts revolve around 're-invention of the wheel.' However, in more lucid intervals we recognize that significant gains have been made in eliminating the territorial imperatives which were terribly prominent during the first two years of our development." Dr. Rieke had publicly expressed his approval of the branch concept, "gave assurance of its inherent academic credibility," and stated to Reed that the Regents and the administration at KUMC had "full confidence in my integrity." Wichita had been given some leeway in recruiting its own faculty, and its departments were "essentially autonomous" from their KUSM counterparts though close cooperation was encouraged.[233] Things were going smoother on that front.

While keeping one eye on those generic issues, Reed and his staff paid full attention to doing what they had intended to do with the new students as well as they could do it. Students responded well to the extra attention they thought they received in Wichita, and a certain type of student preferred the practicum feel of it to the more hierarchical and academic tone of Kansas City. They also liked the city. Dr. Kent Murray once joked, "Wichita is a nice place to live, but you wouldn't want to visit there."[234] That seemed to be the pattern, as students and faculty hired from outside found Wichita much more attractive than its reputation at a distance.

People who had participated recalled that it was "a tumultuous time on the Kansas City campus." There was extreme student distrust of the administration in these last years of the Vietnam era, a large controversy over civil rights, and a fundamental suspicion, even hostility, between students and faculty in Kansas City as well as in Lawrence. Students, therefore, "viewed Wichita as a source of tranquility," a sort of "peaceful kingdom" by contrast where they could pay attention to their career goals without distraction. They were, the student recalled, "like a private in the army," not questioning the system at Wichita much, but interested in working hard and learning and attracted by the opportunity for hands-on experience. Wichita was less a big, crowded, metropolitan area than Kansas City, and KUSM-W was less hierarchic and militaristic than KUSM, "more collegial between residents, students, and faculty." The Interphase was a welcome break from the "nose to the grindstone sessions," and a chance to reflect on what it all meant with the faculty and even with the dean, formally or informally.[235]

The niche of KUSM-W was a compromise for some. Dr. Robert Manning recalled that it was regarded in Kansas City as not a place for heavyweights, but rather a "second tier where people went who could not get a real job in an academic center."[236] However, Wichita was attractive to some philosophically as well as practically. As Dr. R. Lawrence Sifford put it, "Medicine is a human experience and very complex." And that complexity was not just intellectual.[237] There were faculty who had been in traditional medical schools, had been uncomfortable with some of their limitations, and liked the Wichita take on things precisely because of its clinical and mentoring emphasis. Even the lack of bench research was sometimes seen as an opportunity for clinical research by those who saw the best place to do research as "on the front line where the patients are." There was direct responsibility and accountability.[238] The concern, of course, was to avoid a medical school that was a sort of trade school where the student result was limited by how experienced their mentors were and how well they could communicate. In a medical world, where there were 2,000 brain-specific regulatory proteins and over 4,000 different classes of drugs with trillions of possible combinations for individual patients, one's specific educational experience would soon be out of date, and it would be critical whether the student had learned to learn, and to investigate independently—a skill that was at base academic.[239]

All that was in the mix and in the challenge as the school at Wichita grew. In the fall of 1974, Reed and Dominic reported that the Interphase feature was working well, giving students a better appreciation of the roles of doctor and patient, the biology of aging, homosexuality, the dynamics of dying, and a number of other topics. All the while, they said, the more traditional aspects of medical education were being done well. Reed was much concerned that KUSM-W be unique, but not too unique. It had to do what it was born to do, but it had to be a legitimate school of medicine also, and a creditable part of the University of Kansas School of Medicine.

"The major challenge to the WSU Branch," Reed wrote late in 1974, "is to develop a tradition of excellence in a medical education program and to encourage our students to take advantage of the various patient care opportunities, which a city like Wichita provides. All of this must be accomplished in the face of probable fiscal constraints."[240]

Chapter Five

Outreach

Early in 1974, Dr. Joseph Dominic authored a piece called "New Beginnings: The Wichita State University Branch, Kansas University School of Medicine." The school, he wrote "grew to reality in an environment consistent with changes occurring in medical education around the country." As such, its innovations were not so much revolutionary as evolutionary. Courses in medical ethics, aging, human ecology, sexuality, and clinical process were not so unusual any more. Nor were family practice clerkships, which had the virtue of "correlation and integration among all the medical sciences." Some of the "problems, political vicissitudes, strengths, and weaknesses" of KUSM-W were unique to Wichita and Kansas, making it impossible for it simply to borrow another model. Therefore, as it struggled to "authenticate itself," it did so along certain lines for which there was little precedent. The curriculum was designed to produce doctors who were "more preventative and problem-oriented in diagnosing illness, more efficient and expert in sorting out and providing the most effective forms of treatment, and more sensitive to the human conditions in which illness resides."

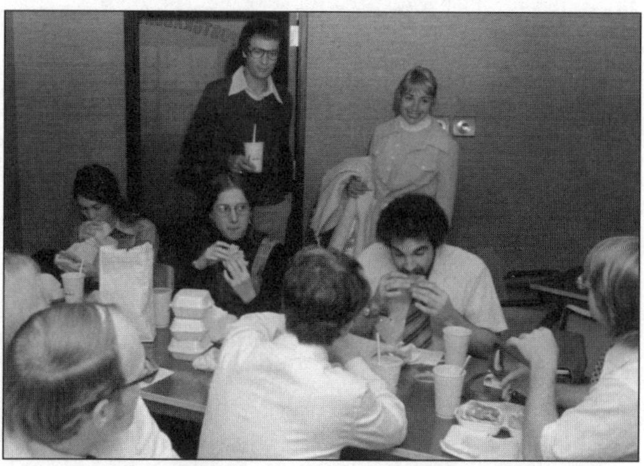

Joseph Dominic, Ph.D. (in doorway) overlooking a group at Fairmount Towers.

There were five required clerkships at Wichita in 1974. Surgery and medicine clerkships occupied ten to twelve weeks each, pediatrics and obstetrics and gynecology were eight weeks, and psychiatry was six weeks. Each discipline used a newly prepared curriculum guide that specified goals for each segment of the course as well as giving reading lists and self-study material. By design, there were not yet required clerkships in family practice or community medicine. The first class of fifteen was divided into three groups with three clerkships in progress simultaneously. In hospitals, students were under the supervision of members of the faculty and senior house staff and were assigned patients for whom they assumed various degrees of responsibility. They were required to participate in daily teaching rounds and to attend seminars and special topic conferences.

When students first arrived, they experienced something called "Introphase." The focus there was on personal goals and communications problems, and it was led by a professional in human relations. Between clerkships, they went to "Interphase" sessions. In these latter sessions, they met away from the hospitals "in an environment conducive to temporary deceleration and eclectic inquiry." They watched films, and were involved in discussions and simulations "designed to provide incentives for broadening their capacity for integrated learning, and for adjusting emotionally and intellectually to the growing complexities of medical practice." For the first class, one of the Interphase sessions was conducted by the director of the Sedgwick County Public Health Department and was called "Medicine and the Community." Another was on homosexuality and was led by two homosexuals who focused on "behavior pattern myths." For the first six months of training in Wichita, students spent time assisting a physician in his or her office. Later they had the option of working with a specialist, engaging in research, or working with a community service agency. After completion of their five required clinical clerkships, a four-week preceptorship was required. This might be served anywhere from a private office to a mobile health clinic. Faculty assessed students and students assessed faculty. "The kinetic nature of these programs," Dominic wrote, "requires constant attention to detail and frequent evaluation. It also requires that the students be self-motivating to the extent of taking advantage of the multiple learning environments at their disposal. Above all, it requires constant supervision by faculty to insure that the goals of each program are being accomplished, and that the various needs of our students are being heard and satisfied."[241]

Reed was confident of his ground, and hoped to stick with implementing it for a time before making too many changes. But change was in the air in these years. One event of 1974 was the creation by the

University of Kansas of an allied health program. Wes Sowers, writing to Chancellor Dykes, noted that a number of legislators were concerned "with what seems to be a significant deviation from an agreed concept in respect to developments in the field of medical education and training." When the legislature approved the bond issue for KUMC, "many of us felt that this carried with it an implied agreement that the development of health-related professions including certain nurse's training would be concentrated upon at Wichita State University." The proposed new title for KUMC, "College of Health Sciences and Hospital" seemed to Sowers "redundant, verbose, and inappropriate."[242] But it happened, thus throwing another wrench into Reed's idea of developing CHRP at WSU and integrating it with KUSM-W. An architect was appointed in the fall of 1974 to design a new building on the WSU campus (it would eventually be named Ahlberg Hall) to house both CHRP and KUSM-W.

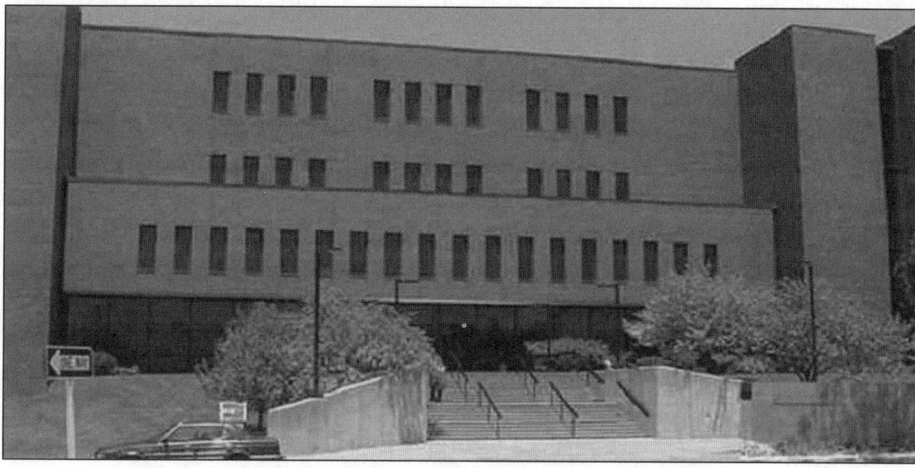

Ahlberg Hall on the WSU campus.

However, the relationship of the two and the relationship of KUSM-W to WSU and its campus was still in doubt. Another issue was the creation of a practice corporation in Wichita. This was related to the campus location issue. "I wish we were going to be closer to the medical community," Reed wrote in October 1974, "but from a political point of view, this simply is not possible; nonetheless I have some concern about the propriety of trying to launch a professional practice corporation in a building on a university campus. For the most part, the students so far seem to believe all of the 'action' is in the hospitals and not out at the medical school administrative facility."[243]

In addition to these "big picture" challenges, there were a large number of more specific "problems for solution," Wichita growing pains as it were, that Reed negotiated about first with Rieke, and then with his successor Dr. David Robinson, who served as acting Executive Vice Chancellor for Health Affairs at Kansas City when Rieke departed in June 1975. Accreditation for the school of medicine in Kansas City depended upon approval of the Wichita operation. But problems had to be solved—diplomatically and carefully—so as not to offend vital local constituencies, namely the Wichita physician and hospital communities. KU must, Rieke said, maintain a "low profile, low-keyed approach of general persuasion." The doctors and hospitals "must be assured that they will not lose their autonomy and independence." The state, however, was demanding a voice in operating Wichita's hospital-based, graduate/resident training programs, since it had invested over $1 million in them so far. An *Eagle* reporter observed, "Reed admits he is walking a tightrope, but he believes the time has come for action to firmly establish the branch."[244]

Rieke and Reed worked out a series of goals for Wichita in the fall of 1974. These included plans to: develop a more functional table of organization for KUSM-W; more accurately define the role and relationship of its Department of Family Practice to its other teaching departments as well as to family practice graduate education programs; complete, formalize, and implement provisions for the professional practice group; concentrate on establishing with CHRP an "interdisciplinary program emphasizing the importance of interpersonal relationship between physicians—patients and physicians—allied health personnel"; continue to improve Wichita's outreach capability; establish a postgraduate medical education capability to serve clinical associate faculty and other physicians in the area; recruit additional "academically-oriented FTE [full-time equivalent] faculty members"; and resubmit a funding request for an associate dean and possibly other faculty administrative positions for support from federal funding.[245]

Rieke reported in November on the visit of the accreditation team to Wichita and provided an expanded list of things to do. The team was impressed "with the supportive and prosperous Wichita community," and the clinical resources there. "They thought that you, as dean of the branch, were a highly skilled diplomat who was giving very effective leadership." Hospital administrators seemed to trust Reed, as did the administration at WSU. The accreditation team saw the involvement of WSU as a strength, particularly the faculty talent that was available in biology, chemistry, and engineering. Ahlberg told the team that he was not interested in a four-year medical school at Wichita, and that it was "educationally and economically non-viable." However Rieke reported that an aide had told him he thought Ahlberg might have a hidden agenda on this. The team was impressed by the department chairs and the large number of volunteer faculty but noted that this kind of enthusiastic volunteering would probably not last long.

Rieke recommended some changes at that point. For one thing the divided loyalty of Reed to WSU and to KU would continue to present difficulties. The team was "convinced Clark Ahlberg had no intention of losing you from WSU," but that issue must be resolved.[246]

Other changes outlined in 1974, however, proceeded. Rieke thought there should be full-time chairs for the departments of surgery and obstetrics and gynecology, as the part-time faculty there created the same divided loyalty difficulty. There was a need for written and detailed memos of understanding between KUSM-W and all the agencies with which it interacted. The financial arrangements were too loose. The school should find teaching faculty in pathology, radiology, and anesthesiology, and perhaps create a department in basic and behavioral sciences. There should be a written agreement between Presidents Ahlberg and Dykes endorsed by the Board of Regents about the use of a new building on the WSU campus for CHRP and KUSM-W. And finally some philosophical issues needed to be better defined. Was KUSM-W the same or different than KUSM? If it was different, how was it different? Their relationship should be more carefully defined and "the chairmen at Wichita need to be reminded that they ought not to drift away from interacting with their fellows here in Kansas City." The school at Wichita, Rieke emphasized in several contexts, could not be accredited by itself, nor could the school in Kansas City. "Rather, Kansas has one school of medicine and it either will be accredited or it will not be."

In this case it was accredited, fully. "You should be very proud and pleased, Cramer!" wrote Dr. Rieke. "I certainly am, for your effort has led to accreditation of a larger medical school, which has a branch that is only the second one in the nation to have a fully approved program in which an entire segment of the education to the M.D. degree [*sic*] is offered. My warmest congratulations and good wishes to a one time 'plumber' turned first rate academician."[247]

Perhaps one way of resolving the dual loyalty problem was the attempt at this time to promote Reed to a post that would tie him exclusively to KUMC in Kansas City. In April 1975, a KUMC search committee notified Reed that he was being considered for the position of executive vice chancellor of the medical center, the post that Rieke was just then vacating. Reed declined on the grounds that others were better qualified and that KUMC could use him better as the dean at Wichita. Also, the dean at CHRP at WSU had recently resigned and Reed felt a responsibility to WSU to continue to help with that program.[248] He did make a suggestion about the type of person who should have the post of vice chancellor. "From a parochial point of view we believe it is essential that this individual . . . have a sensitivity and respect for community-based clinical programs. One of our ongoing frustrations is the lack of understanding of how the branch must operate on the part of several KUMC clinicians and administrators. This person should be supportive of the branch to the degree that he would recognize that it is not possible to mold it into the same form as the typical health science center."[249]

Reed did have a title change when in September 1975 he became a vice chancellor at KUMC, now called the College of Health Sciences and Hospital. Press reports quoted Chancellor Dykes to the effect that Reed would be "an integral part of the administrative team." But he not only remained dean at KUSM-W, he also retained his half-time position as Vice President for Health Education at WSU. The change in title did, one reporter thought, reflect "the stability, maturity and excellence of the now accredited Wichita Branch."[250]

KUSM-W worked hard through Reed for considerable autonomy. Reed emphasized that he and Rieke had agreed that he, Reed, would report to the executive vice chancellor at KUMC, but that the faculty at Wichita would "have linear responsibility to me." Wichita would recruit its own faculty with concurrence from the executive vice chancellor. The Wichita faculty would develop its own curriculum objectives to be approved later by the KUSM faculty. Its clinical teaching modules would be different than those at KUSM and it would perform its own student evaluations. KUSM-W departments would be "essentially autonomous" from their KUSM counterparts, although close cooperation would be encouraged.[251] Reed debated with Dr. Robinson, Rieke's replacement, about what Reed called "manipulation" of Wichita's budget at Kansas City. He expressed "utter chagrin" at KUMC transferring funds without telling Wichita or explaining why. "It does not seem at all proper that the Branch . . . should suffer because of what appears to be inadequate budgetary controls within the Med Center. . . . We can't tolerate many more such fiascos."[252] Robinson corresponded with Ahlberg about Reed's salary, as everyone agreed that he was under compensated relative to other deans of regional medical schools, and that contributed to the idea that Wichita was not quite a full member of the group. WSU and KU were still splitting Reed's salary.[253]

Reed continued to push the same program agreed to by Rieke when Dr. Robert Kugel became Executive Vice Chancellor for Health Affairs at KUMC in April 1976. A list of items to be discussed between Reed and Kugel included: "He should have a pretty clear picture of how we are organized. . . . We probably should make it known that we do not intend to 'cheapen' the academic titles at KUSM by asking for 'special' favors to tenure and promote our people from the traditional concerns of the faculty at K.C." But, the internal memo added, "We need to discuss what 'semi-autonomous' means."[254]

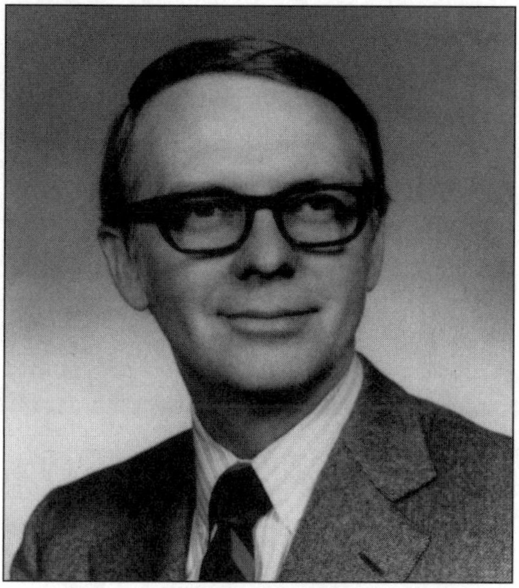

Robert Kugel, M.D.

The Wichita faculty tried to show what it meant in practice. They were not trying to compete, Reed said. "We put it together in a little different way. . . . We haven't gone off into the wild blue yonder to try and reinvent the wheel in the wrong way. There's still only one school of medicine in Kansas." But the 2,200 beds in Wichita gave different opportunities for the second class of twenty-seven and the third of twenty-nine. Dr. Dominic emphasized, however, that it was a complete program, "It's not as though our students are sitting around with family physicians, just learning how to give injections and fix skinned knees."[255]

They worked hard on local implementation through 1975 and 1976. Early in 1975, Wichita began developing a presence at the small, nearby town of Harper, Kansas. The idea was to operate a clinic at Harper as a private practice as well as a means to instruct KUSM-W students.[256] That operation went into the Board of Regents budget for Wichita for fiscal year 1976.[257] The Karl T. Wiedemann Foundation, which had done much for Wichita medicine, granted KUSM-W substantial money in 1975 for instructional resources, student travel, and faculty attendance at national meetings.[258] An anonymous local donor came up with a $100,000 gift to be distributed as Reed saw fit.[259] An arthritis care unit went into Fairmount Towers early in 1975.[260]

The "town-gown" problem continued to fester and be addressed. Local doctors were not eager to have state influence in their practices. "Involved," wrote the local press in a study of the matter in 1975, "is the complex issue of meshing a formal university medical program into a more loosely structured community-based system of medical education and care." KUSM-W depended on private physicians and community hospitals to be successful and, in 1975, the extent of that commitment became clearer. "We all raised our hands," said Reed. "But none of us really knew at that time what it meant. Now we do."[261] One doctor commented, "You have to gear down for the medical students, like talking to the PTA, and it's just not as much fun."[262] Most, however, enjoyed it and excelled at it. In 1976, Dr. Farha of KUSM-W won the Thor Jager award from KUMC for excellence in teaching. Dr. Dennis Ross, an internal medicine resident at Wesley, won the vice chancellor's award for distinguished teaching by a resident, while Dr. Bobby Webster at Wesley and Dr. Cullen Thomas at St. Francis received certificates of recognition in that category.[263] There were other encouraging statistics about the first class. Seven of the first eleven scheduled to graduate from KUSM-W announced plans to remain in Wichita in post-graduate residency programs. That was exactly what had been the hope.[264]

The school became ever better integrated into the community. Jan Riordan R.N., for example, did a workshop on breastfeeding in the fall of 1975 co-sponsored by the KUSM-W Department of Pediatrics, the Kansas LaLeche League, and the Kansas Bureau of Maternal and Child Health Care.[265] That year the school established an internal newsletter called *The Branch Log*, so that it had its own publicity organ independent of the *WSU News* where its goings-on had been previously reported. Dr. Roberts appeared on television that year concerning a controversy over the birth control pill.[266] He was most active in lobbying for reform in Kansas malpractice award laws.[267] Residents at Wesley formed a Daniel K. Roberts Society to promote excellence in teaching, research, and practice of obstetrics and gynecology.[268] Dr. Guthrie that year led the Kansas affiliate of the American Diabetes Association group on a backpacking trip in the mountains of Colorado. He was gaining a national reputation for his work with diabetes and held seminars with his wife around the country.[269] Dr. William Eckart, a clinical associate of KUSM-W had an international reputation in forensic pathology and in 1975 was elected president of the International Association of Forensic Sciences.[270] In 1976, the pediatrics residency for Wichita, a major goal of the Department of Pediatrics, was accredited and approved.[271] Working lunches began to be held with the staff at the *Wichita Eagle* to ensure that medical reporting was more fair and accurate in the city.[272] Workshops sponsored by KUSM-W were frequent, in topics ranging from family and youth, to respiratory therapy, to gastrointestinal bleeding, to reproductive care.[273] Beginning in 1974, KUSM-W sponsored a physician-community day (later called Health Day). In 1975, more than 120 people from forty-eight communities attended. In 1976, there were 275 people from seventy communities. There were lectures by the KUSM-W staff on the advantages and disadvantages of rural practice. The mayors, city council representatives, and members of chambers of commerce and civic clubs were instructed on how to recruit doctors directly out of KUSM-W, and the day in

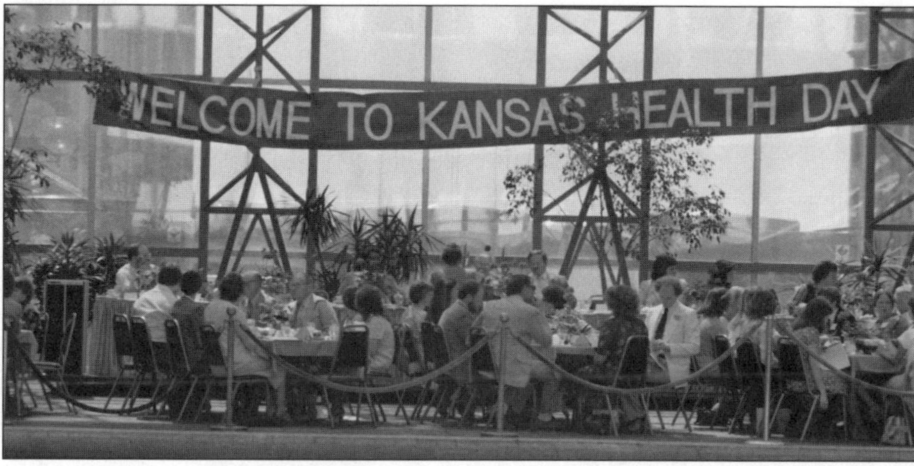

Health Day began providing physician recruiting opportunities in the mid-1970s.

Wichita gave them a chance to make direct contact with physicians in training and to present the case for locating in small and medically underserved towns in Kansas.[274] Dean Kortge was most active in meeting with medical societies, and not only sponsoring workshops in their towns, but in the case of Salina and Hutchinson, also developing residency programs.[275] Seven area hospitals subscribed to Kortge's mobile education program for small hospitals to train service staff in the same van that had been used for hypertension screening. The van, by the fall of 1976, was visiting hospitals in Anthony, Harper, Attica, Caldwell, Kingman, Marion, McPherson, Winfield, and Wellington once every three weeks. It provided four, one-hour sessions with programs on audiovisual tapes for as many as sixty people at a time.[276] In 1977, there was a pediatrics outreach program added, including a baby clinic at various towns in western Kansas run by Dr. Vernon James of the KUSM-W staff.[277]

This excited Kortge, as he and doctors flew to some places and drove to others. To him, breaking down barriers was "fun," and so was working in rural Kansas, both to train people there and to help those communities recruit doctors. However, he had the feeling that it was not a priority with KU, and he was not as diplomatic in expressing frustrations about it, as was Reed. Increasingly, he thought there was a "deeply felt division between us and them," and that KUSM-W was perceived as a "burr under KU's saddle." At Wichita the staff was "very passionate" about the outreach but felt that the Kansas City people were only tolerant of it. In addition, KU, Kortge remembered, was determined in the late 1970s, to "definitely put their *imprimatur* on the branch."[278]

Part of the tension here may have had to do with the management style of Chancellor Dykes. Dykes did visit Wichita, he was interested in its progress, and he played a far more active role in supervising day-to-day details than other chancellors had or that most in the office would. He wanted to unify the University of Kansas, had enormous energy and tolerance for detail, and admitted, "Some accuse me of being a micromanager." He was, he said, "deeply and actively involved," though at times it might have been better for him to "keep his nose out," as his interest might be misinterpreted. Robert Docking, whom Dykes thought was a "wise and effective governor," had brought the new chancellor to his office at the time of his appointment to the KU post and had asked him to take a stand and be the spokesperson for the synergism that should exist between the academic and the medical world. Dykes started spending one day a week at KUMC, which was unprecedented, and gave the KU financial officers control over the budget and central administration of KUMC as well as KUSM-W. He created an office of general counsel at Lawrence to which all other lawyers in all parts of the university system reported and who, in turn, reported to Dykes. Dykes felt that a "more tightly knit and more unified whole" was important academically and politically and was what the Kansas Board of Regents wanted.[279] Dykes had a strong personality, strong opinions, and an effective and wide reach. Whatever issues concerning Wichita's role in relation to KUMC and KU remained unresolved would be brought to a head by the Dykes administration and resolved one way or another. If it led to crisis and change, so be it. But whether he was a benevolent dictator or not depended on one's location in the system and one's point of view. Certainly he was a University of Kansas loyalist and an administrator with a style of central control. Insofar as either of these characteristics was unattractive to people at KUSM-W, the Dykes administration would be accordingly unattractive, too.

Certainly Dykes would not follow a policy of "drift," or "benign neglect." Dr. David Waxman, who became executive vice chancellor at KUMC in 1977, recalled of these years that administrators did not need constant direction, but did have their marching orders. There were certain things that went on at the university "and I knew what they were and did not make any attempt to change them." These policies were based on shared goals for education, and the "fact that there is a university holds it all together is my feeling." If the Wichita faculty were under pressure, so, Waxman was quick to point out, was the KUMC faculty, and the reason was that these were times of "remarkable change." Despite it all, "It ended up all right," Waxman emphasized. "It did not collapse."[280]

In the meantime, however, there was constant adjustment, adaptation, or polite conflict. It seemed sometimes that in Wichita it was what one new faculty member there called "sky is falling" times.[281] In actuality, there was a lot of movement and compromise on all sides.

Take, for example, the consideration in 1975 of a name change for the Wichita school. That was abandoned because of "Ahlberg's sentiments."[282] However, the debate over it reflected some of the tensions. The proposed change was from "Wichita State University Branch of the Kansas University School of Medicine" to "Kansas University School of Clinical Medicine at Wichita State University." This, by no means, eliminated WSU from the title, but the old title might imply that WSU was a branch of KUSM, while the new one, it was thought, "maintains the visibility of both institutions without demeaning either," while better stating the mission.[283] Ahlberg recalled that the current title had been approved at a meeting in Morrison Hall in September 1971 and he had a "strong feeling" it was still good. He and Reed, Ahlberg pointed out to Chancellor Dykes, had spoken to many groups in Wichita emphasizing that they had no desire to create a separate freestanding medical school in Wichita, but also emphasizing that Reed needed "a degree of independence to develop a program focused on turning out physicians to practice medicine and to build an integrated allied health professions and undergraduate medical education program." They had had assurances "that the undergraduate medical program would not be a mere extension of the University of Kansas School of Medicine in Wichita, but, indeed, would be something different and responsive to the health needs of this region," while strengthening WSU in the areas of allied health, biological, and physical sciences. WSU could support KUSM-W "without in any way threatening the University of Kansas's control of the medical branch." Did Dykes share this view? "Frankly," wrote Ahlberg, "I have come to feel that that is not desired by you and that, indeed, there is no longer any role for Wichita State University in the undergraduate medical educational program. I hope this is not the case, but that is the impression that has been conveyed to me."[284] Dykes apologized for any misunderstanding, backed away from the name change, and pledged continued cooperation in the collaborative effort.[285] Clearly, however, what seemed like a discussion of a minor name change had involved a good deal more than that.

Reed was restive about certain things. He thought the title "Branch" was "denigrating," and so did his faculty.[286] He remembered that, while he was invited to participate in faculty meetings in Kansas City, these meetings were always held at 8:00 a.m. Kansas City regarded him as someone from Wichita who needed to be "watched," while Wichita regarded him as an officer in contact with Kansas City who needed to be "watched." Wichita financial supporters and city boosters wondered where his loyalties lay. Also, the local faculty was hard to manage by definition and was filled not only with its own brand of suspicion, but also with its own ambitions. Drs. Roberts and Farha had practice "empires" and large incomes, while

Drs. Voth and Guthrie, for example, also department chairs, did not. None of them was as used to taking direction as parts of a large organization.[287] Roberts and Farha, Dr. George Dyck of the Department of Psychiatry remembered, were people who had their own power base, as other chairs did not, and "there was no escaping that the dean could not really tell them what to do; they had to be persuaded."[288] There were struggles about the private practice clinic that developed within KUSM-W and about who was creating that income and to whom, or to what departments it would go. Kortge with his Ph.D. in history, his "scraggly beard and cowboy boots," did not necessarily mesh easily with even the Wichita physician community, not to mention the more distant establishment in Kansas City. People had their eye on the ball they thought was being pitched to them, and had a hard time seeing the big picture. There were, Reed remembered, "lots of games played by these people," and managing it all required "serendipity" at the least.[289]

"It is not infrequent," he wrote Dykes in March 1976, "that my efforts to keep up with the unfolding of the events on the Kansas City campus are frustrated by the ambiguity of my administrative positions and my remote location." His current example was that he had learned of proposals to establish another clinical branch in Topeka by reading the minutes of a faculty assembly meeting. "It is not that I am ignorant about the need for additional clinical training space or educational personnel in the immediate future. That is a formidable reality for all of us. Nor do I feel so naïve as to ignore the political expediency of such topics. However, my sense of 'things as they are' tilts toward severe anxiety when I consider the possible uncontrolled friction that such discussions and eventual action might cause." All had worked hard to "soften the lines between previously factious north-south elements." Now it was Reed's turn to worry about losing financial support because of competition somewhere else in the state.[290]

To colleagues, he expressed frustration too. He wrote a fellow urologist: "Thanks for your kind remarks about my 'Deaning' or whatever, but I can assure you that much of the time I wish I were back in urology."[291] And to a faculty member in Kansas City, he wrote that he had considered taking a supportive letter from the man to bed with him at night as his "blanket." Reed said no one could know how much he regretted that "the Kansas City faculty are so 'hyper' about the Wichita campus." He had said many times that there was no interest in forming a separate medical school, but maybe the desire to get more autonomy from the Lawrence campus was interpreted that way. "Be that as it may we find ourselves in an almost continuous state of siege because some of the people up there *assume* that we are attempting to break away from the parent institution." All Reed asked was "that there be an understanding of our need to be slightly different."[292]

Chapter Six

Sea Change

The doubts and worries were perhaps an intimation of the change that was coming. The next two years were an extended pivotal moment for KUSM-W, a sea change in its culture and administration marking the end of the experimental, maybe at times a little whimsical, early phase of its development.

Perhaps it began with the appointment of Dr. Robert Kugel as Executive Vice Chancellor for Health Affairs in April 1976. Kugel and his successor Dr. David Waxman were not interim or bridge officers, but permanent parts of the KU administration. As such they were perhaps viewed by Chancellor Dykes as proper instruments to make reforms he was interested in making in the relationship with Wichita.

In his opening address to the faculty, Kugel said there were those who wondered why he would want the job in such a time of crisis. His answer was that KU had a fine history and tradition and there was a chance to build on it. He was proud of the "solid accomplishment" at Wichita. The administration there had "done the necessary planning and carried out their plan in a bold and imaginative fashion." Kugel expressed great sympathy with the goals of KUSM-W, especially that of humanizing medicine, and of being "concerned with compassion for the ill, comfort for the weary, and understanding for the anxious and distraught individual in our midst."[293] However, the machinery there could use modification.

There was an immediate administrative change at Wichita. In June 1976, Reed hired Dr. Richard Walsh, who had been working with rural health programs in New Mexico, as associate dean of KUSM-W, with the official title of Associate Dean for Administrative and Community Relations. His job responsibility was primarily "internal management and operational matters," with perhaps 30 percent of his time devoted to remote community programs. Reed sent him the KU Faculty Handbook.[294]

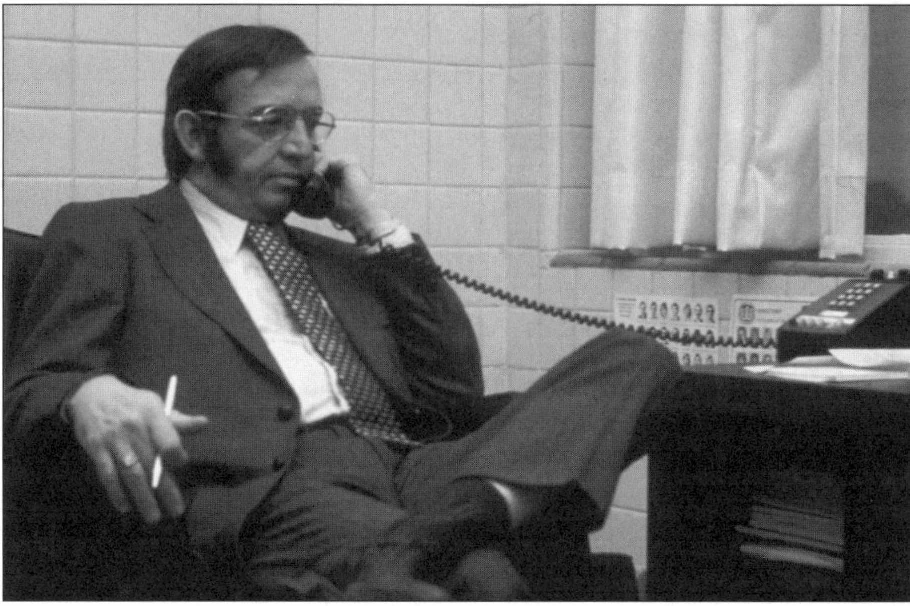

Richard Walsh, M.D.

Walsh was no "button-down" executive recruited by a headhunter. He had been a surgeon in the Korean War and in Silver City, New Mexico, for sixteen years.[295] His background was appropriate for the job and his style and ideals (casual and passionate) would seem to comport well with the institutional culture at KUSM-W. There was no doubt Reed could use the help that an associate would provide. Walsh was to focus on academic affairs while Reed specialized in administrative activities and "the field of community relations."[296] Still, with the Walsh appointment, for the first time there was an "outsider" in the Wichita administration, not part of the founding group, not a native Wichitan, and doubtless representing to some an attempt at tighter KU control.

Certainly it did not mean that Reed was withdrawing. He wrote Dykes in August that he used to spend 70–80 hours a week in his urology practice, but had more free time then than he had now. It was offensive to have the press questioning how faculty and administration time was spent, as it had been doing. Reed said when he added it up he came up with a 150 percent time commitment with at least a 125 percent reduction in pay compared to his private practice days. "If you believe a surgical procedure would be appropriate in this case," Reed concluded his letter, "I hope you will keep me in mind as I have not completely divorced myself from the practice of urology and possibly could help the 'cause' with some form of surgical intervention involving the genito-urinary tract."[297]

For his part, Walsh was able to see the situation from an outsider's perspective, and there was virtue in that. He could see, for example, that there was still some support in town for a separate medical school, and that it was a potentially dangerous situation. He concluded early that Chancellor Dykes was the "ultimate political creature," and "not the kind of guy who would tolerate any competition whatsoever." If Dykes got wind of any lingering idea that there might be a transition at some point to complete autonomy, Walsh thought it would have been "death by a thousand cuts" to anyone connected. He could see also that there was a town-gown problem, and that physicians and hospitals were concerned about competition from the KUSM-W practice corporation. He felt that one of his best accomplishments in the KUSM-W administration was to collect data to show how miniscule that competition really was and present it in a speech before the Medical Society of Sedgwick County. Walsh's experience in rural medicine also applied. Based on that, he thought some of the Kansas thinking about rural health care was a dream. He did not think, for instance, that towns that could not afford a John Deere tractor agency and a Ford dealership could afford a doctor, whether KUSM-W provided Health Day recruiting events or not. He thought regionalization of rural health care was the answer.

So there was a new slant and style and, as Walsh put it, a "tremendous shift in relationships." He remembered Dykes telling him "get those people happy," but that there was no particular plan for doing it. He found the weekly meetings he attended at Kansas City and Lawrence "chilly" at first, but felt that, as years passed, KUMC seemed less threatened and more accepting.[298] The more difficult transition in relationships was no doubt in Wichita. Stepping into the shoes of such a beloved local figure as Reed, even in a limited way, could not have been easy.

There was awkwardness in institutional relationships and leadership style, which this move was a start at addressing. Reed and Dykes were both strong leaders, but different types of leaders in charge of different types of organizations with different goals.

Reed was a *primus inter pares* (first among equals) type whose situation forced a style of coordination by persuasion and a good deal of latitude not only for talent, but for ambiguity and eccentricity. He had the creative and maybe wooly-headed animus of an entrepreneur in a start-up but perhaps lacked some of the qualities needed in the manager of a large or mature organization with more to protect than to develop. He said in 1976, "The pursuit of medical education and the practice of medicine is neither a dispiriting undertaking nor a continuously delightful adventure." Living was, to him, "the integration of all aspects of existence into a well-ordered, meaningful experience," of which technical training was only a part.[299]

Dr. Robert Hudson of KUMC put the challenge humorously, but accurately, in a 1980 speech. "Running a successful academic institution," he wrote, "is more in the nature of zookeeping than sheep ranching, and I use the word zoo here in its strictly positive aspect. Certainly managing a sheep ranch is easier and less complicated than running a zoo. The sheep are docile and comfortably alike, they accept their regimented existence without complaint, give up their fleece periodically and predictably. But a successful zoo requires a good deal of attention to individual differences. Many of the animals therein are independent-minded, temperamental, and some are even downright ornery. But it is this very diversity, which makes the zoo superior to the sheep ranch in terms of the function of a university. If all the animals in a zoo were made to act like sheep, by whatever means, the job of management would be infinitely easier, but the zoo would no longer serve the function for which society created it."[300]

There was evidence that Reed was tiring, especially of trying to juggle his two roles. He wrote Dr. John Breazeale at WSU in the spring of 1975: "Quite frankly, John, the personal satisfaction and rewards of the two positions I occupy here are, in themselves, not sufficient to compensate for the psychic–physical trauma and the inordinate amount of time I have found necessary to devote to the various tasks associated with the two titles." The two positions, he said, "are no longer 'all that fun'; rather they involve rigorous, time-consuming, serious, hard work."[301] He expressed a similar view to Dr. Ahlberg. He was fairly thick-skinned, Reed wrote, and not easily depressed, but there was constant worry in taking issues maybe all too seriously. He wondered if "the relationship between the two of us wouldn't be better if you and Chancellor Dykes got someone else in this job who is more academically oriented to avoid ongoing conflicts. . . . It simply seems that I don't know how to function as an administrator responsible to several line officers without getting 'crosswise' with at least one—who is a good friend; life is pretty short for this, don't you think?"[302]

More than anything, Reed wanted clearer definitions. The legislature seemed to consider KUSM-W either as an "expensive toy of someone," or as "a real vexation and think we should go away." Wichitans were divided. "Many Wichita people think we are WSU. Others think we are KU but ought to be WSU—Most don't know what we are." Reed continued to make his lists of thing to change, but often his ideas were unrecognizable by the time they were implemented.[303] This did not surprise him, but it frustrated him.

Dykes was no sheepherder, nor was he without strong entrepreneurial instincts. But he did have more of a business model of the desirability of centralized policy and enforced hierarchy. He was sympathetic to the dilemma of Reed's double appointment. "You may be assured," he wrote him in 1975, "that I will understand the sensitive environment in which you work."[304] But Dykes was interested in "establishing precedence for what will follow in our Wichita Branch," and therefore wanted to "organize and structure the programs in the most productive fashion."[305] The search for truth and beauty required a functioning and secure organization, and what the prayer book calls "singleness of heart."

For all the respect that Dykes clearly had for him, Reed, with his high-level contacts around the state and his not disloyal but independent agenda for Wichita, could throw a wrench from time to time into the model of a well-oiled machine. Dykes spent time in Wichita. He developed his own constituency downtown and among the faculty, and it was not necessarily the same as Reed's. The goal was not to suppress the creative juices in Wichita, but to control the institution there and coordinate it with the "one university" to which Dykes was committed. He wrote Wichita attorney John Eberhardt, for example, in the spring of 1975, that a recent appearance of Dykes and staff at a meeting in downtown Wichita had as "part of the hidden agenda" to "demonstrate that the University of Kansas is capable of retaining control over the medical branch and that there should be no consideration whatsoever to the creation of a second medical school." He added that he intended to do his utmost to see "that no further medical expansion, no law school expansion, and no graduate education expansion occurs at Wichita State University. We already have too much higher education in Kansas, and we certainly don't need another school that tries to emulate the University of Kansas."[306] While emphasizing to the local press that cooperation between KUSM-W and the University of Kansas was very good, he also pointed out that the KU School of Medicine was seventy-six years old and its branch was a comparative infant.[307] There should be no question of lines of authority. "It is essential," he wrote an assistant, "that we become deeply involved in all matters pertaining to the branch. . . . Our presence will help cement the 'one medical school—one university' concept. This is one of our important goals and we must do everything possible to bring it to reality."[308]

Given those differences in personal approach, and given the impossibilities for any one person of the dual appointment Reed had, it was perhaps inevitable that the tenuous "co-existence" of KU, KUMC, WSU, CHRP, MSSC, the Wichita business community, the legislature, and the hospitals would not last in its original form. The first graduates of KUSM-W received their diplomas in May 1975. The classes behind them were filling. There were forty students in Wichita in 1976, and it was estimated that there would be fifty in 1978, or 25 percent of KUSM's total class of 200.[309] The AMA, in the spring of 1976, accredited the school so that its postgraduate courses for doctors were eligible for AMA Category One continuing

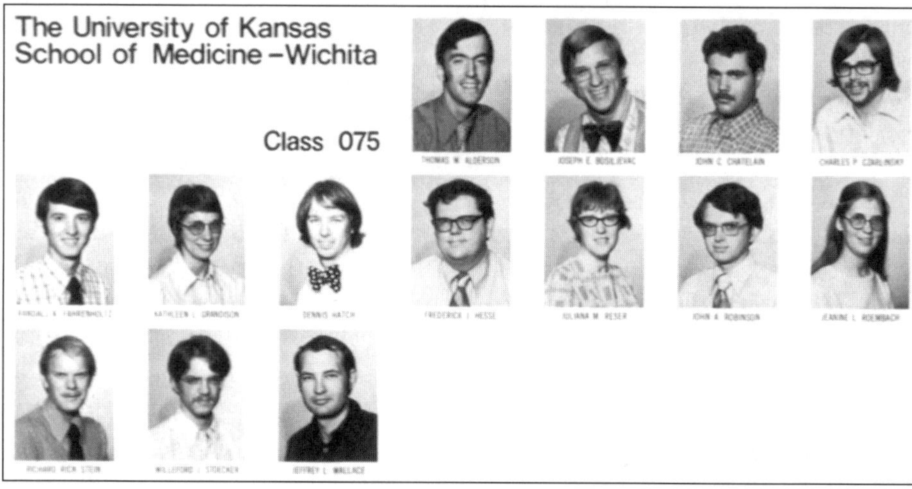

KUSM-W's first class graduated in 1975.

education credits.[310] It was obvious that the Wichita division of KUSM was established to stay, and that no temporary arrangement would any longer suit. The Walsh appointment, therefore, was the opening move in a series of administrative events, rapid by institutional standards and complete by 1978, which radically changed things at KUSM-W. First, Reed separated from WSU; then KUSM-W separated from WSU; last Reed separated from KUSM-W. There was no question that a significant part of the initiative for these events was with the University of Kansas.

Step one was Reed's resignation of his post as Vice President for Health Education at Wichita State University. Formally this was to take effect in February 1977, but Reed informed Ahlberg of his decision in the middle of December 1976. "This note is a most difficult one for me," he began, "but write it I must." He explained that his decision was based on circumstances arising from a meeting of department chairs from both campuses, and that he wanted to inform Ahlberg before the rumor mill got going. It should, Reed said, simplify relations between KUSM-W and WSU's CHRP.[311]

The faculty meeting to which Reed referred was a long and strenuous one. Dykes and Kugel had arranged to meet with state legislators at the "Shocker Club" at Wichita State about the relationship between WSU and KUMC, certainly sending a strong message that either the KUSM-W should itself move to clarify it, or officials and Lawrence and Kansas City would do it on their behalf.[312] There was a late afternoon session between KUSM-W faculty and President Ahlberg, and then a meeting of the executive faculty.

That group advised Dr. Kugel in Kansas City to make Dr. Reed a full-time employee of KUMC. It voted unanimously to recommend changing the name from WSU Branch of the University of Kansas School of Medicine to University of Kansas School of Medicine-Wichita. This name change happened the next June. Dr. Farha first made a philosophical motion that Chancellor Dykes might himself have made: "It should be recognized there is but a single faculty of the University of Kansas School of Medicine with one campus in Kansas City and a second campus in Wichita." There was a two-hour discussion about that one and about "how the matter of governance between the branch and KUMC might realistically be carried out." Several substitute motions were considered and finally one passed that recognized continuing differences. It stated that there was one school of medicine but "two divisions of the faculty," and "each of these divisions has different environments unique to itself." The motion added: "These two entities need both independent and interdependent functions."[313] Immediately after Reed's resignation at WSU a joint task force formed called the "University of Kansas, Kansas City-Wichita Liaison Committee."[314] It was to define how the two campuses would interrelate in the future while remaining committed to the idea of decentralized decision-making.

Reed saw also from that meeting that there was a "rift" between KUSM-W and CHRP. He did not think this need be a "donnybrook," but he did see that his dream of close coordination between medical doctors and the allied health professions was not shared widely by physicians in the community or his own faculty.[315] There had regularly been questions too from the accrediting group about "the validity of the person responsible for branch administration having a similar responsibility at another institution."[316] For personal and political reasons, therefore, it seemed a good time to end the dual role. He wrote about this time in fact that he was "inordinately pleased" to finally have only one job.[317]

Reed worried particularly about the reaction of Wichitans. He told Ahlberg he thought trying to explain the change or allowing speculation to run could create "an unhealthy situation for both of us."[318] Certainly there were some local backers who felt betrayed and blamed both Reed and Ahlberg for what they regarded as giving in to the enemy. Larry Jones, chief executive of the Coleman Company, wrote President Ahlberg that the change of status for Reed "seems based on agreements that are either fraudulent or superficial," and appeared to him to be "an opportunistic power play" by KU and maybe by Reed. Jones thought Reed's move had caused "anger and resentment" among local people that would damage the further development of KUSM-W. It was just another example, he thought, of the subordination of the realities of Wichita's size and success "to the personal and provincial interests of the University of Kansas." Wichitans had thought the medical branch was "a creature primarily of

WSU," but now it seems WSU was being left aside. "I'm not sure which camel's nose has entered the tent, but I'll call it Archie."[319]

Reed wrote Dykes reporting the faculty vote and his decision. He explained that he simply had to get rid of the "ongoing concerns of Kansas City and Wichita campus faculty regarding my loyalty to the parent institution." It seemed that "future intercampus relations, in large part, hinge on a clearer definition of my dual roles,"—something that Reed had said more than once before. KU's creation of an allied health program complicated things further. "It is no longer possible for me to maintain personal integrity while attempting to relate to potentially competitive allied health and nursing faculties on two campuses." Eliminating the "WSU acronym" from the name would be helpful too, Reed thought, in improving faculty recruitment, faculty and student institutional identification, and federal institutional grant affiliation.[320]

Dykes was sympathetic and supportive. "I know these next few days will be tough for you," he wrote. "I'm convinced we should stand resolute on our plans to come with the university full time. If we don't force the issue now, it will continue to be a problem for the future. Perhaps our discussions with Clark will generate a breakthrough. Please be assured I'm prepared to stand with you come what may." Dykes thought that because of Reed's "great stature" in Wichita, his friends would understand that this was not a move to harm the branch but "rather it will help assure its fullest developments. . . . Hold firm and good luck!"[321]

Certainly, there were some immediate changes in the way KUSM-W was administered. Yet the general experimental and somewhat casual atmosphere of the place remained. Dr. Anne Walling visited in 1977. She was moving from England and joined the Department of Family Practice in 1981. On this first 1977 visit, she was both impressed with Dr. Walsh's lack of a necktie and the fact that a woman carrying a baby was so welcome and respected at the institution. However, she was totally unimpressed with the physical plant and vowed she would never work there.[322] RoxAnn Dicker began working in 1977 with the outreach program. She reported both

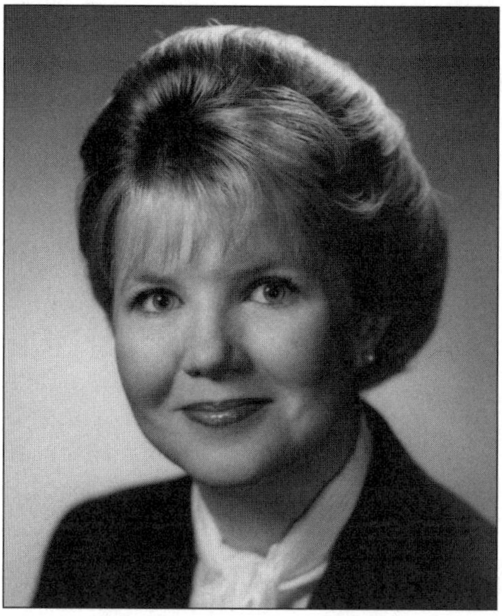

RoxAnn Dicker, Associate Dean

to the dean at Wichita and directly to Kansas City, a new twist. Her impression was that she could do with outreach what she could raise the money for, but that those programs, so basic to the early years of the institution in Wichita, were never going to be part of the regular budget under more close control from Kansas City. She said that Dykes had an entrepreneurial spirit and that some of her programs, including creating a Department of Public Health for the State of Kansas, ran into somewhat more of a headwind actually from WSU "our natural ally" than they did from KU.[323]

The next stage of the revolution, or evolution, was complex, but decisive. It involved the official change of the name of the branch to KUSM-W and a move to an ill-prepared E.B. Allen Hospital and away from the WSU campus building already in process of construction. Symbolically and physically, this represented a complete break from any future relationship with WSU, formal or informal, agreed or understood.

The name was a formality, although clearly the WSU administration, which had been against even the rearrangement of the title, could see the writing on the wall when all mention of WSU was excised. But that only confirmed what the move away from the campus affirmed.

The move was not to better quarters. E.B. Allen Hospital, in the condition it was in when the move was made in July 1977, generated a universal feeling of disgust by those who had to office and work there. This was true even by contrast to the minimal environs at Fairmount Towers. Reed reported to Ahlberg that the move went fine, but that it was a "come down" from the nice furnishings at Fairmount Towers. It did seem more to resemble a medical facility, and he thought parachute material might be used to hide some of the damaged ceiling and unsightly plumbing. He admitted, however, that "I tend to have certain 'Polyanna' concepts."[324] There was a strong smell of urine, alcohol fumes, and vomit. There were birds in the building, no air-conditioning on the third floor, little parking space, and the physical layout was anything but suitable for the use to which the building would now be put. There was not even a secure tenure there. Sedgwick County still occupied most of the space, leasing KUSM-W only a little over 28,000 square feet of the 50,000 the school thought it would need by 1981.[325] There was still a title problem with the land, KUSM-W continued looking actively for an alternative site, and it was by no means certain that the county would ever be willing or able to sell or lease the entire E.B. Allen building to KUSM-W.[326] Only Dr. Reed seemed happy with it, working away at his office in a former operating room under the bare overhead light as though it was just another adjustment.[327] Dr. Farha said that with the minimal budget and such a horrible facility the thing became "boring. There is no intellectual curiosity. Guys will leave."[328] One of the women who tried to add a little color to the place could only describe it as "pathetic."[329]

The move was a shock to the administration at Wichita State University. Late in 1976, ground had been cleared on the campus along 17th Street for a 62,500 square foot building to house CHRP and what was still then the "WSU Branch."[330] Reed did express concern that the 22,687 square feet allocated to KUSM-W in that building would be inadequate, but adjustments could be made.[331] In fact, it was not immediately clear that the move from the campus was irrevocable. There was publicity that the move to E.B. Allen was temporary, pending the completion of the new campus building in 1979. It was only in December 1977 that the Kansas Board of Regents decided that the medical school should remain at E.B. Allen rather than move to the Health Sciences Building at WSU. The official explanation was that plans to share the building with CHRP had proved unfeasible due to the continuous growth of both institutions.[332] The real reasons, however, seemed to be more administrative than physical.

Reed got wind of the change in plans for the WSU building in June, just before the move to E.B. Allen. A legislative study committee visited Wichita, toured the E.B. Allen site and the campus, and intimated that it did not feel there was a need for the campus building. Reed wrote Marlin Rein, chief legislative fiscal analyst in Topeka: "Marlin, it would be a catastrophe if by any chance some kind of action would be initiated to stop that building at this point in time for a variety of reasons, not the least of which would be the local flag over my resigning from WSU. There isn't a single person in this area who would believe that the branch or I didn't have something to do with it, and I'm sure it would close us up in short order."[333] Dykes agreed it was a "sensitive political issue," in Wichita, but wrote a legislator that the Wichita faculty liked E.B. Allen and the campus building would not do. He did not, however, want to "do anything that would concern those of you in the Legislature or create problems for us or for our friends at Wichita State."[334]

Rein himself, reflecting years later, said that Dykes recognized that a move into that building on campus would create a perception in Wichita of an association that had been informal and which Dykes did not want to perpetuate. Wichitans had "a high sense of ownership of the school in Wichita," but this had no formal justification. "I don't think outside of Wichita," Rein said, "anyone saw it [KUSM-W] as having any relationship to Wichita State University, other than a shared deanship and the location on the WSU campus." But given that location and given Reed's recent dual role, it was only natural that people should assume WSU was a major player. Said Rein, "People were never going to understand the reporting lines as they should unless they separated them entirely"—unless and until "you broke the chain that tied it to Wichita State." The events bringing about the separation, Rein remembered as "a little painful to watch," but he had no doubt some such moves were necessary and desirable.[335]

Dr. George Platt who was the head of planning at WSU received the news without warning that the new building would not have its intended use. In fact, the architectural plans had to be significantly changed to transform it into what, in a fine irony, became Ahlberg Hall. Physicians in Wichita had pressed for a location on a main street rather than in the interior of the campus to give them and patients easy access, and much about the layout of the building was directed toward its medical use. Both he and Ahlberg were, as Platt put it later "extremely disappointed when the venture collapsed." The move away from the building did not just leave a building to change, but was the end of a dream for Ahlberg and the state's only urban university. It was, Platt said, an "element of our relation with the community which would have been a great experiment and which we were all pushing for."[336] Dr. John Breazeale, who had been involved since the first tentative planning in 1969, was upset and disappointed, also. Ahlberg was an astute enough politician, Breazeale said, to have suspected the change for some time, but it was the end for him of a "great and appropriate opportunity" for his university.

Perhaps there were some who thought that was the end of major changes. It was not. In March of 1977, Dr. Richard Walsh was named acting dean of KUSM-W. In August, he became dean.[337] In September, Dr. Kugel resigned at KUMC.[338] In October, Dykes invited Reed to apply to replace Kugel as executive vice chancellor in charge of KUMC and Reed refused.[339] In April 1978, Walsh resigned as dean at Wichita.[340] Reed moved back into the deanship. The next month, Reed resigned as vice chancellor of KUMC and dean of KUSM-W.[341] Walsh was convinced to withdraw his job applications and stay on as Wichita dean.

As always, it is the details more than the bare statement that fascinate. Reed was becoming increasingly frustrated with the administrative coordination with KUMC, or lack of it. He wrote Dr. Joseph Meek, who was director of Health Care Outreach at KUMC in January 1977: "I hope you do understand, Joe, any implication of 'anger' subtly expressed in such communication from us does not in any way imply that it is directed to you as a person. Our problem is a continuing one." Reed thought it was lack of identification with the parent institution and lack of identification of channels and line authority for various programs. "And often try as we do to perform in the proper way, it never appears to be quite right or we find that instructions have been issued someplace else but have never been given to us; consequently, we may seem to perform in a vacuum." There were too many cooks working at the same stove, Reed said, "and one doesn't know what all the others are putting together."[342]

Walsh's appointment as acting dean was a response to that. Reed would remain a vice chancellor at KU and continue to represent KUSM-W in legislative, regents, developmental, budgetary, and strategic planning matters. Committees would be appointed by Kugel to find a permanent dean for Wichita. Reed wrote his faculty that the administrative alignment had been anticipated for some time, and that there would be some changes in Kansas City also to eliminate a perception of mixed or dual authority over allied health there. It would, Reed said, "make it possible to implement a more cohesive and effective governance-administrative system than would otherwise be possible." He, himself, would remain "closely involved," but could specialize in broader matters.[343]

Some of these broader matters clearly worried him. He wrote Dr. Stephens in Huntsville that he was frustrated that the community supporters in Wichita were not unified. "I have had high hopes that they were indeed getting together about the graduate medical education thing only to learn . . . that the hospitals are so fearful of each other and paranoid about the branch that it looks like the consortium which we mentioned on the phone is not likely to come about simply because the hospitals can't find a way to deal with it." Under those conditions, what would a strong head of the Department of Family Practice do, Reed wrote, "but shuffle papers?"[344] He wrote another friend: "We haven't found the right 'button' to push that would place the medical school on the same footing as the 'regulars' in the community."[345]

Dykes again sympathized. "We know the nuances of your complicated relationships in Wichita place heavy pressure on you personally and professionally." Dykes talked with Ahlberg early in April about Reed's status, and reported that Ahlberg seemed more amenable than before about Reed's coming to KU full time. Ahlberg, however, thought the matter should be discussed with the Kansas Board of Regents, and with that Dykes disagreed. "I dislike this since it has the potential for controversy but also because it sets a bad precedent. As you know, the Regents have heretofore given us a rather free hand in making administrative changes and in handling administrative matters."[346] Reed wrote back: "I have from time to time prepared all kinds of lists of reasons why the change in my relationship is important to the well-being of the branch, however, at it now stands I'm not sure if these would have relevance. Help!"[347]

There was pressure on Reed about his friendship with Ahlberg, and he was thinking of his long association with WSU, going back to his student days there. "I presume there may be times in the future," he wrote Ahlberg that spring, "when your patience with me will be tried to the utmost (if I decide to stay with it); however, I want you to know that it will never be my intent to deliberately create situations that are inimical to your personal well-being or that of WSU." No matter how it might appear "I could never develop the affection for KU that I hold for my own school." He had to "play the game," he said, "in order to remain part of the team." But this did not mean his heart was in it. "So I reiterate again only because it was my perception that it couldn't work any other way did I make this painful choice. So you see, to a certain extent, I'm still something of an idealist though my commitment to this philosophy has been tested on a number of occasions."[348]

Dykes naturally saw Reed, wherever his heart lay, as now in the KU camp. He understood Reed's concern about innovation in Wichita. "As you suggest, the branch can contribute most to medical education by being unorthodox, by having some latitude to try new and unproven programs." Dykes would support Reed, he said, within state rules and regulations and he would try to protect Wichita's portion of the budget. Reed's salary was now $56,000, up from his initial salary in the mid-30s, and Dykes expected that "we will be able to use your talents and abilities in a number of important KU activities in Wichita and elsewhere. By and large, these would transcend both the branch and the medical center."[349] That last Reed resisted. He wrote: "I suspect that we would both agree that any overt movement on behalf of the University of Kansas in the Wichita community would be ill-advised. . . . Feelings are running very high . . . and it seems prudent that we not press such matters at this time." He thought that as it was, some of his activity in Wichita on behalf of KU would get back to Ahlberg "which I suspect will not please him at all."[350]

Actually Reed was having some doubts whether the split with WSU would really solve his personal difficulties or the problems of KUSM-W. He wrote to Sister Bernadette, chief executive officer of St. Francis Hospital, in June 1977, noting that he was "fascinated" by the possibility of working there. "However, in light of the recent unfortunate flap about my going full time at the University of Kansas, I feel that I must stay in the system for the present or there would be those who would feel that I was running from the problems that have been created, and for which I must stay and rectify."[351] At that point, he left the door open to renew discussions about a different job in the future when circumstances might change.

There continued to be publicity and personal contacts that left Reed feeling that people in Wichita did not trust him and thought him disloyal to the community. He wrote Larry Jones that the issue was "emotionally laden for me," but that he had done what he thought was best for health care in Kansas. "I regret that my actions are considered circumspect and that you believe I have 'used' the people of Wichita for ulterior purposes." The state's interests were broader than those of WSU.[352] To Dwight Button at the Fourth National Bank, Reed admitted that he was not defending himself much. "It is not my style to fight fire with fire."[353] To Dykes he wrote: "One really needs a crystal ball in this business Archie. Attitudes and principals affecting us seem to slip around."[354] He also wrote Terry Scanlon: "This hasn't been the most pleasant period of my life."[355]

Still he made his list of goals as usual in July 1977 for the next fiscal year and sent them to Dykes. The first one was to assist in restoring KUSM-W "as a recognized prestigious health-education institution." He would put together a local advisory council, finish the search for a permanent dean and a chair of the Department of Family Practice, and work on the "ambiguous" positions of Drs. Farha and Roberts.[356] Dykes communicated back that Kugel was not working out and that Waxman would replace him in Kansas City.[357] The announcement of Walsh as permanent dean of KUSM-W shortly followed.[358]

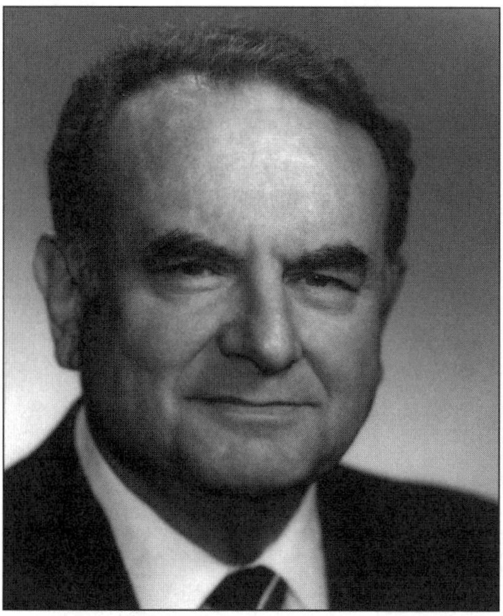

David Waxman, M.D.

Dykes was enthusiastic about Waxman as Kugel's replacement in the job of executive vice chancellor at KUMC, but Reed expressed some doubts about how satisfactory that might be in the long run. Waxman, he thought, was not involved enough in state and national educational activities. Perhaps the position of executive vice chancellor could be eliminated and replaced with a kind of head of operations not expected to represent the entire system externally. Reed implied that Walsh's appointment as dean would relieve Reed of some tasks "and I am willing to take on others."[359]

Apparently Chancellor Dykes took him very much at his word on this. He asked Reed to serve as university advisor on legislation pertaining to health education.[360] Then he asked Reed to consider becoming executive vice chancellor of KUMC himself. This was the second time the offer had been made, the first being in 1975 when Dr. Rieke had left that post.

Reed again declined. He did not wish, he said, to threaten the calm now in effect in Kansas City, and Waxman seemed to be doing well and be accepted well. Reed felt his managerial style might not be acceptable to the faculty in Kansas City and was certain that his lack of academic background would be a handicap. He also was sixty-two and, at the moment, felt older than that. He could support KU best, he said, by staying in Wichita.[361]

On that front, Reed was satisfied that the break with WSU was complete and the transition to being comfortable at E.B. Allen was well along. "As negative as all this may sound," he wrote Dykes, "we have yet to have had a visitor who has not confided that they could see no possible way for us to ever move back to campus, out of the facility we are presently in." Therefore, he and Lorene Valentine were working on the budget with the assumption that there would be no more drastic facility changes. They would just have to do expensive remodeling so that they could get office space, for example, for the four faculty members who were in the fall of 1977 "farmed out" to hospitals for lack of room for them at headquarters.[362] Dykes agreed strongly. He was worried about an "apparent lack of awareness in Wichita" of the school's affiliation with KU. Because of its former location on the WSU campus "many people have viewed the School of Medicine in Wichita as part of Wichita State University, with which it has never had any official connection."[363] Dykes, however, did defer to Reed in allowing KUSM-W to be the only exception among the divisions of the university in not using the KU seal on its official letterhead.[364]

The next administrative shocks came in the spring of 1978. Dr. Walsh began seriously looking for another job in April. He was leaving Wichita with regret, he said, but in discussions with Reed "it has become apparent that there is indeed only a single administrative position here, and the confusion created by having two decision makers in an institution of this size is detrimental."[365]

Actually, the number of decision makers seemed to be on the rise. Walsh appointed Dr. William Reals in March as Assistant Dean for Research, Development, and Planning.[366] There was a local advisory committee formed in April.[367] Walsh, as dean, immediately suggested hiring an assistant dean for academic affairs.[368] Reed noted to Waxman, "As you well know, tables of organization are often developed to accommodate certain kinds of individuals who are available rather than saying what you think Utopia should be."[369]

There was some internal tension. At a faculty meeting held February 28, there was an extensive discussion of what were called "crucial problems" facing the school in the immediate future. These, including space allocation, had "precipitated a sense of urgency." The faculty thought the needs of the school were not understood by the administration or the legislature and "expressed the belief that the present system is nonfunctional and becoming more so daily." The chairs and program directors threatened to approach the KU chancellor directly with their grievances. They feared that they would have to reduce the number of students at Wichita or discontinue the program there entirely. There was not enough time to devote to teaching, much less to research, and an unsatisfactory student-to-faculty ratio. The budget was inadequate to retain current faculty much less to recruit more. After five years, the volunteer faculty was becoming tired of volunteer service and would need to have more support. In addition, where was KUSM-W? There was no certainty that E.B. Allen would continue as its home, and the "indefiniteness of the physical" future made it hard for the school to project stability. "The medical and hospital administration entities are oriented to fixed long-term commitments as a security base which they have worked to establish; they do not perceive [KUSM-W] as having any permanency, consequently they are reluctant to 'throw in with the University.'" There was anxiety about accreditation, since one of the requirements was that there be "a connected series of educational activities controlled by a full-time faculty coordinated by the administration and integrated with the program of the main medical center." The Wichita faculty doubted that they could show that. They thought that the departments of psychiatry, internal medicine, and pediatrics would have to be relocated at hospitals. They concluded that the "immediate and future growth of the Wichita program is at a standstill."[370]

Reed worried. The accreditation people would require some evidence of academic research. Yes, Reals was on board to push that, but there was little time and it would be hard to show.[371] In fact, when legislative committees visited, they wanted to see that Wichita was not engaged in research and therefore was not in competition with Kansas City in facilities or support.[372] That was incompatible with what the accreditation team wanted to see. Reed wrote Dykes that he hoped the faculty minutes conveyed "a sense of urgency." Dykes had reassured the faculty which, Reed thought, "did much to reduce the level of paranoia" that existed not only among the executive faculty group but among the support staff." He would do all possible to "keep the boat at an even keel," and to accomplish Dyke's goal of keeping the present faculty for at least a year.[373]

But amid all this, Reed kept having his personal credibility problems at WSU and around Wichita. To a person of his character that was particularly distressing. In April, he had to respond to an article in the WSU student newspaper. It claimed "KU Medical School Skips Out, WSU Asks for State Help." Had KUSM-W committed some sort of crime? There had been space problems at Fairmount Towers and difficulty getting a long-term commitment, not to mention KU's goals. Reed wrote James Rhatigan at WSU reaffirming his loyalty to Wichita State and reaffirming that "I have certain responsibilities, of course, as an administrator of the University of Kansas which have nothing to do with my own emotions." He much regretted the "innuendos and occasional outright allegations that have emerged regarding my 'desertion.' I can assure you that all of this has not been satisfying or conducive to digestion."[374]

On May 2, Walsh wrote Waxman that after discussions with the chairs about his resignation, the upcoming accreditation visit and the future of Wichita he had decided "despite my personal anxieties" to stay on.[375] Two days later Reed wrote Dykes that he did not wish to be reappointed as vice chancellor for KUSM-W. "Over the past several months," he wrote, "I have given considerable thought to my effectiveness as a member of your administrative staff. I have reluctantly concluded that I am not serving the university appropriately."[376] Dykes accepted, noting briefly that Reed would be "sorely missed."[377]

Actually, yes and no. As is so often the case in such matters, Reed's resignation covered the fact that he had been asked to resign.[378] His position at KUMC was eliminated when he left. For all his frustrations with the situation, he was not comfortable abandoning the school in the state it was in then. And having taken so much heat from his Wichita constituencies for "selling out to the enemy," it was hard not to be able to stay long enough to prove his point. But Reed was a realist, and he had predicted from the time he left WSU that he might very well not retire as a KU employee. He had an excellent sense of himself and a humble perspective. His virtues as a person were many, but no doubt he had some shortcomings as an administrator and man of action. Hamlet, the thinker and deep human being, put the dilemma of the humanist as reformer well in noting that "the native hue of resolution" could be "sicklied o'er by the pale cast of thought," causing "enterprises of great pith and moment" to "lose the name of action."

Dr. Walsh wrote a friend that he had been approached to serve again as dean and had agreed. "There are many challenging jobs to be done here and who could resist that."[379] The school had grown. It started in 1974 with fifteen students, fifteen paid faculty and staff, and 100 volunteer physicians. In 1978, it had ninety-four students, 175 paid faculty and staff, and 275 volunteer physicians.[380] But growth was not an unmixed blessing. It would be some time before all the "challenging jobs" could even be sorted out much less addressed. Reed's departure was the end of an era for KUSM-W with no certainty about what the new era might be. To say that it was an anxious moment for all would be an understatement. Dismissing Reed, said one faculty member, was "like shooting the Easter bunny."[381]

For Reed himself it was, in some ways, a relief, but he did not feel immediately relieved. The Reeds had a series of granddaughters staying with them and his ninety-four-year-old mother had died May 26. And, although he had arranged to go to work at Wesley Hospital in July, he was temporarily out of a job. "So, all in all," he wrote Dr. Stephens, "this hasn't been the greatest spring we've had. Nevertheless, I know that we will eventually make it okay."[382] So, he hoped, would his institutional child in Wichita, the so-called "stepchild" of the University of Kansas.

Chapter Seven

A Precarious Balance

For accreditation purposes KUSM-W did a self-study in 1978. Surely, too, it was an appropriate time to take stock of where the institution was then. The study noted that the school had multiple constituencies, internal and external, local and distant. The student needed "the development of his educational skills and his ability to eventually function as a well-rounded physician." The faculty needed resources to accomplish its educational mission as well as those needed "for personal growth academically and professionally." There was another Wichita constituency external to the institution proper in the physicians and hospitals of the community of Wichita. Then there were the distant needs of the medical center at Kansas City and the University of Kansas at Lawrence. "Their expectations are primarily meeting standards of excellence and representing the institution well in the community its serves." Even more distant, but vital, was the external constituency of the state government, whose expectations for the production of doctors for rural areas "continue to bear upon the performance of the Wichita branch." The mission needed to remain "vital and current."

In 1978 the most critical difficulty with a constituency was the relationship of the medical school to the community of Wichita. "The separation of the medical school and WSU," the report confessed, "was extremely traumatic for many people in the community." It was predicated on "ongoing conflict between intrastate rivalries," but the two universities had "delayed dealing with a number of community relations problems," and so these continued to fester. There had also been "a small undercurrent of anxiety" in Wichita about KU's "taking over" Wichita medical education. Partly these things were endemic to a community-based school. As such, it was important "that we constantly re-define the relationship between the community physicians, volunteer faculty members, and the medical school."

The school was in a growth mode, and it was not time for spare finances. In that regard, the report concluded, KU was "quite generous" with its Wichita division. Because Wichita faculty generated less income than was usual with medical school faculty, the percentage of support from the state was unusually large. Perhaps eventually as the number of faculty and the number of full-time academic faculty increased, the teaching workload might decrease, and there might be more time for both research and practice within the school. Meanwhile, on matters such as curriculum and faculty tenure, practices at Wichita and at Kansas City were becoming more standard and more similar. E.B. Allen was being quickly upgraded and the hospital-based clinical facilities, always a strength, remained outstanding.[383]

One change that was ongoing was the growth of the University of Kansas School of Medicine-Wichita Faculty Practice Association. In fiscal year 1974, the first reported, this organization had three stockholders and generated income of $19,240, all from pediatrics and psychiatry. The next year it earned over $76,000, and added internal medicine and family practice. Fiscal year 1976 created $210,340 in income. By 1979, there were twenty stockholders, thirty-one income generators, and the yearly professional fee income was over $750,000.[384] In 1978, Dr. Voth was concerned that ambulatory care activities were still inadequate to provide either adequate income or a "predictable patient flow for student education."[385] Still, progress there was slow but sure, and certainly too much activity in this field would exacerbate the town-gown relationship problems.

Clearly there remained doubt about the relationship with KU, and about the variation in types of faculty. Dr. Richard Walsh wrote in February 1978 to a colleague in New Jersey. He said: "The governance relationships between the branch and the main medical center are of considerable significance. . . . It is difficult to deal with the adjustments of a community setting. . . . It becomes exceedingly difficult if the faculty at the main branch does not feel they have any ownership in the branch and views it as an unwanted child whom they have little interest in supporting and nurturing."

Internally, Walsh noted, two of the department chairs at Wichita "have control of a large segment of practice within the community in their specific departmental areas" and had large incomes. This created a number of problems "none of which have become near crisis proportions but have caused concern for the primary loyalty of these chiefs of departments." Time and experience had shown that their loyalty to the university was unquestioned and there was no doubt "they have an enormous influence in establishing the school in the community and developing its community support." Still, it required the full-time academic faculty to "adjust their thinking" and this took time. Ultimately, Walsh thought, there would have to be a transition away from such an extreme community-based model. This was partly because "it is really not possible to provide supervision and quality control without full time faculty" and partly because the wide variance in model and mission complicated relations with KUMC. Day-to-day operations were complex when "one is dealing with a group of primarily private practitioners who do not understand the disciplines of an academic institution or the hierarchy of an academic power structure. The private practitioner has a much greater degree of autonomy and decision making and feels himself impossibly restrained within the decision making parameter of a university hierarchy." Thus, despite the great advantages of the community-based model, it carried problems with it.

Obviously, too, in the immediate aftermath of Cramer Reed's departure, an aura of him, for better or worse, remained. There was stress at the suddenness of the change at the top and anxiety about its import, given the rather long tenure and massive influence this single person had. It was almost as though Emerson was literally correct in saying that an institution is only the lengthened shadow of one man. Jerry Lessard, who had been the first full-time professional person hired and who left the school in 1979 to pursue a Ph.D., ruminated years later on the impact of Reed's departure. "He was the model of a patient-focused physician and I don't know if he knew how good he was at that." The school, he remembered was "presenting great examples of physicians for students to emulate. . . . That is what drove us and I missed it when I left." Lessard remembered of Reed's departure that "to say we were shocked would be an understatement. . . . All of a sudden your mentor, your leader, the inspiration for your organization is gone." It would have been easier, he thought, to accept Reed's death than "to have him expelled without explanation." There was no ceremony of honor, no liturgy of transition.[386] Change is inevitable and no institution can afford an indispensable man. Still, it was an occasion for much thought within the school and the city.

The *Wichita Eagle* covered the resignation and the aftermath extensively, collecting differing opinions of the future of KUSM-W. One comment was, "There is continued erosion of the decision-making process, plus a lack of teachers, research and financial support." Another said that Wichita was sufficiently reimbursed to run a quality program.[387] A third noted, "He [Reed] has been the guiding light, the driving force, and whatever else it takes to make a thing go." While Reed himself commented, "somebody else may be able to do better," many doubted it.[388]

Dykes, the newspaper noted, had no plans to fill Reed's position. Perhaps he had been placed in an impossible situation that should not be repeated. Certainly the early years had led the school through "some intricate political thickets." Reed commented, "There are no manuals in developing schools like this." Dykes shared some of Reed's frustration in the sense that Dykes had difficulty figuring the direction of the legislature. "It's frustrating," he told the Wichita paper, "to not know whether you're pleasing them or not until something is done." His hope was to establish continuity.[389]

There were, however, challenges there. It was uncertain still whether KUSM-W would remain housed at E.B. Allen Hospital. In the fall of 1978, there was still a serious search going on for alternative facilities, the main candidate being the five-story "East Pike" building at Kellogg and Webb.[390] However, there was also consideration of the former Kapaun High School site at Woodlawn and Central, the southeast corner of 21st Street and Woodlawn, the northwest corner of 21st Street and Woodlawn, part of the Veteran's Administration property, the so-called Blue Goose Medical Building at 3333 East Central, and even a downtown site.[391] "We feel a little paranoid," said one faculty member of this searching.[392] About the only thing that seemed certain was that at last the name became the University of Kansas School of Medicine at Wichita, with all references to a branch or to WSU finally removed.[393]

The *Eagle* thought that at least Reed's departure "leaves a gap in Wichita and Kansas." Reed had become one of the nation's most "respected and influential spokesmen for medical education." And survival of KUSM-W was not enough, the local paper thought. "Replacing the present first-rate institution with a second-rate one would be tantamount to destroying the whole medical school structure for which Dr. Reed and a few others worked so long and so hard."[394]

Dr. C.T. Hagen of Wichita was one of the first Wichita doctors to comment publicly. He wrote Chancellor Dykes in May 1978 that Reed was a treasure. "I am not certain of your knowledge relating to Dr. Reed's unusual ability in his already monumental effort and very significant success in orchestrating the diverse educational possibilities in our city. If you really aren't looking for trouble, you will find some way to encourage Dr. Reed to remain in the system. KUMC's red-headed stepchild 'The Branch' needs all the help it can get from such unusually talented people."[395]

The resignation worried Walsh also. It was important, he wrote, to consolidate support from faculty groups at KUMC and hospital administrators in Wichita "so they do not take contradictory or antagonistic stands." Hospital administrators seemed concerned about the school's longevity and expansion plans.[396]

That view was shared by Dr. Douglas Voth, chair of internal medicine, and someone who minced no words. "There remain," Voth wrote, "gross disparities of exceptions, responsibilities, vested authorities, and available monies," as well as "substantial lack of comprehension by the State of Kansas about what problems we face, what responsibilities we have, and what it takes to carry out our mission."[397]

Larry Jones, president of the Coleman Company, had always been an outspoken supporter of the WSU connection and of the view that KUSM-W was really a Wichita institution in origin and purpose. After Dykes appeared at a Wichita Chamber of Commerce meeting in May, Jones wrote him a long letter. Yes, he had been critical of KU and of Dykes, but Dykes should understand his reasons. "Wichita, since its founding, has been a community with strong pride plus more than a bit of stubbornness and independence. For the most part, it has struggled to its survival and progress with some lack of interest and some obstructionism from the Topeka/Lawrence/Kansas City center of power." It had been apathetic toward state politics and a little provincial, and this seemed another example of those historical failures. KUSM-W had a legitimate mission, but there was fear this was going to be diluted, and that the separation from WSU and the departure of Reed signaled this. The situation in mid-1978, Jones thought, was "balanced precariously . . . between accepting these moves as proper and well considered and a fury about Wichita being denied an opportunity to construct a major university and a complete medical education institution because KU and its supporters are 'afraid of the competition.'" Wichita could "go to the streets politically" on this, and there was pressure to do so. Community spirit was tied to WSU, and WSU deserved a fair shake.[398] Jones later was to run for governor of Kansas, so determined was he that state politics needed reform.

Reed himself recommended against any vindictive behavior. He discouraged Wichita City Commissioner James Donnell from pushing a legislative investigation of the reasons for Reed's dismissal or resignation.[399] He wrote Wesley Sowers, a legislator, that he was not interested in any form of "anti-social behavior." He was concerned for the future of medical education in Wichita and hoped that some of the ambiguity that existed under his leadership could be clarified at his departure. Stability was important to faculty recruitment and faculty recruitment was vital to success.[400]

The media impression of a "grab" or a "war," however, was hard to dissipate. Fred Weaver of the legislature wrote directly to the Fredonia newspaper emphasizing that the school had always been a branch of KU, and that the only real tie to WSU was Reed himself. "Your editorial would lead people to believe that all is lost for some reason you did not explain." Dykes had supported Wichita, the paper's "rather unkind assertion" about him notwithstanding. Wichita's trust was to train primary care physicians, "and nothing has been done to interrupt that cause."[401]

In December 1978, Dean Walsh gave a full-dress speech to the Medical Society of Sedgwick County with the goal of calming any town-gown friction and of emphasizing that KUSM-W was by no means in disarray. His primary emphasis was that the contrast between community-based schools of medicine and others was narrowing as economic conditions changed, and that all medical schools were moving from full-time to what was called "geographic" full-time faculty. This was brought about by loss of the category of poor, indigent patients who used to be captive to the university teaching hospitals, but who now, with third-party and government payers, had their choice of hospitals. It was also brought about by the increased cost of medical education and therefore a requirement that faculty generate income. This had "created the tension between faculties and communities which exists everywhere. This is a fact of life." It was so much a trend, Walsh said, to work in the community and community hospitals that medical education professionals were seeking a new generic term to describe how schools formally called "community-based" really differed from traditional medical schools.

As the other schools were moving toward the Wichita model, Wichita needed to move in the direction of a more traditional model. It needed a core of full-time faculty to meet accreditation standards and to ensure continuity and support "so that medical education does not degenerate into apprenticeship training, uncoordinated, unsupervised, unevaluated." True, there had been a change in the medical community such that the competence of those in private practice was equal to that of full-time academic faculty. But these physicians could provide only isolated hours and that interfered with continuity. Wichita projected an ideal of eighty-two, full-time faculty, but recognized that it could probably not achieve much more than forty, or one for every two and one-half undergraduate students. "It would be a ratio which would meet the national accreditation requirements and would be acceptable to the political economics within the state legislature and, hopefully, to the local community."

But there was fear in the Medical Society of Sedgwick County that the increase in faculty size "will cause the university to take over the medical community and to force change in hospital standards and requirements that will radically change practice within this community." Walsh saw it as his mission to lay those fears to rest. There were nearly

600 doctors in Wichita, he noted, and it was hard to see how forty, full-time faculty at KUSM-W could dominate hospital staffs. It was an "unrealistic anxiety." And there were many compensating advantages to exposing students to practice in an "excellent private practice oriented tertiary care center." These were the ones that the school had always emphasized. "I feel very strongly," Walsh said, "that the attitudes toward patients, the personal involvement, and dedication, which occurs in that atmosphere, is far superior to the more isolated academic sphere which is found within many research-oriented institutions." KUSM-W had less than one-third the full-time faculty that an academic center would require. They needed to practice to maintain competence. As a competitive factor, they were negligible. One doctor Walsh talked to in private was surprised to learn that he personally generated more income in a year than the entire KUSM-W faculty. "Yes," Walsh noted, "we are in economic competition with the members of the community and we do so with both hands tied behind our back." KUSM-W faculty needed to have a practice supporting their salaries and the school, and they needed a permanent and decent administrative headquarters. "It is possible to function in a tent," quipped Walsh, who had been with a M.A.S.H. unit in Korea. "Many of us did that during the war, but it is not desirable or efficient and certainly not stable." It was time to put doubts and fear aside, accept KUSM-W for what it was and should be, and move beyond the entrepreneurial start-up stage of its history.[402]

Reflecting back on it, Walsh felt this speech had more positive impact than anything he did while in Wichita. Having an "open confrontation" with the dissenters in the medical society, he felt, stopped the creeping rumors and got the issues on the table. Walsh collected data and made slides showing that the average full-time faculty member brought in less than $10,000 in patient billings to the school, and that most of the people in the audience paid more than that in income tax. That, he said, "busted the bubble," and the town resistance waned.[403]

A second major concern of Walsh, in addition to the perennial one of relations with Kansas City, was the sparse research establishment at Wichita. It was hard to recruit well-established research people to a new school with limited resources and a non-research culture. "We find ourselves all too often with untrained, but optimistic and willing people, who wish to undertake research work to develop their own career requirements." But Walsh had "serious concerns" about the quality of the research "and whether one may not wind up just promoting scientific dabbling rather than any quality research activities." Funding was so limited that Walsh thought that in research "our future is fairly dim." It might be said, "we are hitting the wrong end of the curve to be starting up a medical school, but unfortunately, ours is not to choose the time, but rather to complete the necessary plans and development."[404] Walsh found the time to get married in the spring of 1979 but otherwise was fully occupied at the office.[405]

That same spring the state legislature authorized acquiring E.B. Allen hospital as a permanent home for KUSM-W and appropriated $1.3 million for renovation. Walsh was delighted, as this would give stability and provide identity.[406] He wrote Waxman that the aesthetic and functional improvement of the building would be key in converting E.B. Allen into the University of Kansas School of Medicine-Wichita, not only physically, but in the minds of local residents and physicians.[407]

The school took formal possession of the building in December 1979.[408] At a ceremony for transfer earlier, there was an unveiling of an oil painting of Cramer Reed.[409] Reed had objected to the painting on the grounds of cost and because "I must admit that I think it is easier to deal with the future than to dwell on the past, so I have a natural inclination to avoid most forms of eulogy."[410] Most, however, thought it was most appropriate that the portrait be one of the first elements of the new decorating scheme. And in some ways the honor placed the Reed administration firmly and symbolically in the "museum" category of the past. Reed himself continued to maintain a low profile on the circumstances of his removal and to support the new dispensation. He turned down opportunities to meet with community leaders and Dykes. He was no longer angry, he said, though disappointed, but did not intend to share details with any but a few close friends. "For the most part everybody in Wichita considers the matter closed and could care less about what I think."[411] He had new challenges and new contributions to make and that, rather than regret, was his specialty.

To cement good community relations and to make the KU presence in town more acceptable, Dykes and Walsh instituted a local fund-raising campaign in the summer of 1979 with a goal of raising $1.5 million through an organization of Wichita leaders. While both recognized it was a "delicate issue," they felt that Dr. Reals, who was well-known in the community would do well coordinating such a campaign.[412] Dykes wrote Paul Wunsch, a leader in the legislature: "As you know so well, it has been a difficult struggle to get the medical school accepted in Wichita, but we believe now that we are well on the way to being accepted as an integral part of the medical establishment there."[413]

Conditions during the renovation phase were perhaps worse than ever. When Dr. Anne Walling started work in the Department of Family Practice in 1981, her impression was of a landscape of "green pipe and tiles." There were few people in the building at any one time, all focused

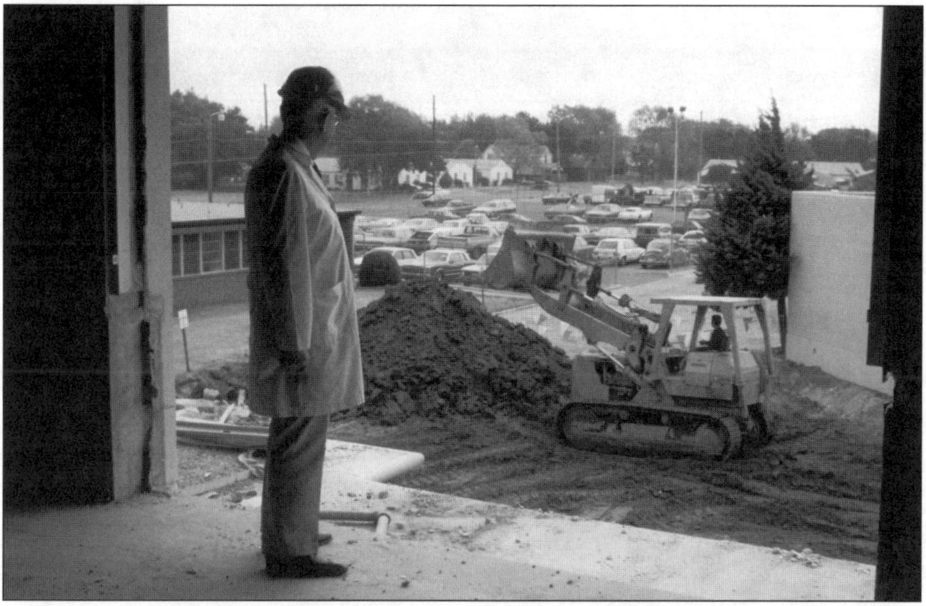

The school underwent dramatic change in the early 1980s.

on developing their own programs, and the sound of jackhammers would have made interdepartmental camaraderie difficult anyway.[414] But prospects for the future looked brighter and therefore patience was stronger. Barbara Delhotal, formerly a freelance writer, was secretary for students in the Department of Internal Medicine in 1980 and 1981. In those days there were still a few lock-up county mental patients in the basement of one wing of E.B. Allen. Dr. Voth and his department staff were located on second floor west and struggled to operate through construction dust. At one point when a new mezzanine was being built, two parts of the school were physically separate from each other. Delhotal had to go downstairs and across a courtyard to make a photocopy. Fire safety regulations were primitive. A staff member of the Department of Pediatrics, also on the second floor, was in a wheelchair and there was talk of how to get her out in case of fire.

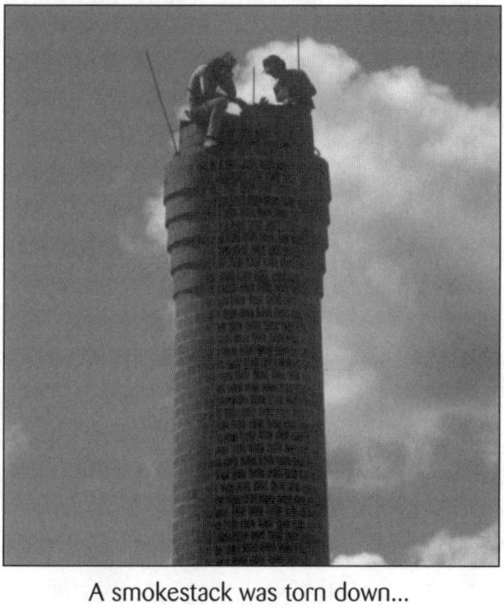

A smokestack was torn down...

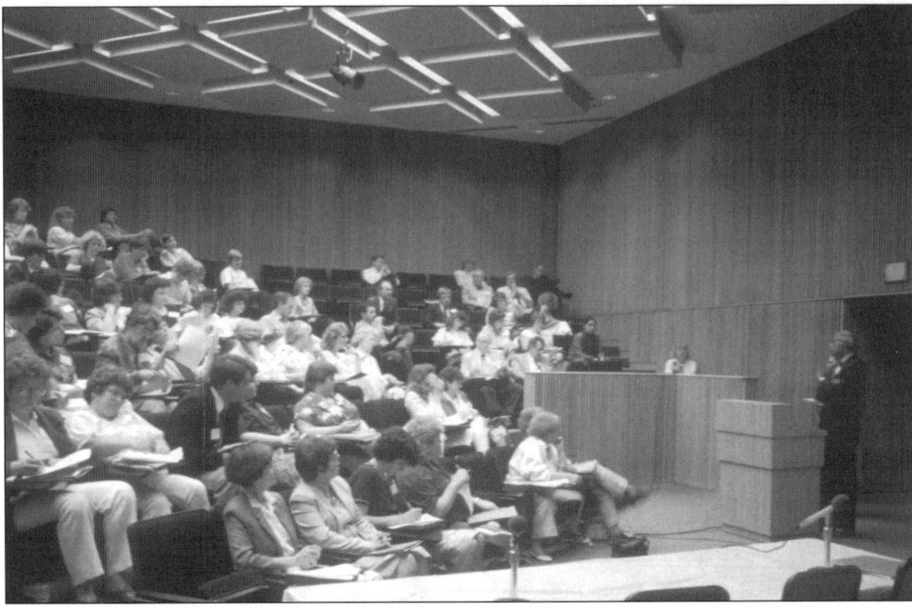

...to make room for the Roberts Amphitheater.

The group decided to carry her if needed. Delhotal remembered the "appalling condition" of things and the "leftover hospital smell." The entire school was gray, including the carpeting and walls, and the women employees particularly made efforts to cheer things up. One Christmas, the employee morale committee decorated the doors. Voth who had a "stern and uncompromising exterior" had his door decorated with a full-sized picture of Darth Vader with the caption "Ho, Ho, Ho." Delhotal's door had a stuffed Mrs. Santa typing on a computer. There were potluck lunches, organized on the spur of the moment with tables sometimes set up in the halls. One of the facilities employees brought soul food once a week, and people gave him a dollar if they wanted some. There was a stained glass class in the basement. There was communication and cooperation, and the school had an "impressive public face," Delhotal remembered, no matter how "ragged" physical conditions might have been. As time passed, Delhotal thought, there was a change that differentiated "a teenaged medical school and a grown up one. We went from blue jeans to a little more dignity." But the blue jean stage had its attractions.[415] "We were all good friends," recalled Dr. David Street, who worked with the surgery rotation, "and it made for a great environment to create a student educational program."[416]

The neighborhood, largely African-American, was closer and more interactive with the school than later when the campus expanded. Vince Marshall, who developed media and communications facilities while using a cobbled together darkroom, came to E.B. Allen once to record a series of lectures on family medicine. The meeting was in the lock-up ward for mental cases and alcoholics in the old annex, and it gave Marshall a "foreboding" feeling to buzz the buzzer to get in and to hear yelling and banging down the hallway. But he put up with that and with the lack of fancy editing equipment and made numerous educational programs on three-quarter inch videotape. Once his Chevette was vandalized, painted with the word "Crips," the name of a Los Angeles-based gang prominent in the crack cocaine trade in Wichita during the eighties. Marshall said that did not bother him. He was occupied with putting up a microwave antenna for distance learning because E.B. Allen had a great high and central location near the hospitals. But it must have bothered others.[417] It made an impression on Dr. Anne Walling, for instance, that many of the KUSM-W staff watched the police one day raid a crack house right under their noses in an era of drive-by shootings.[418]

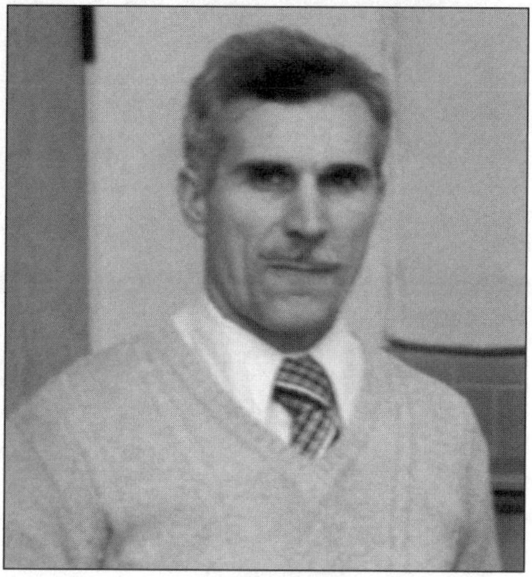

Vince Marshall

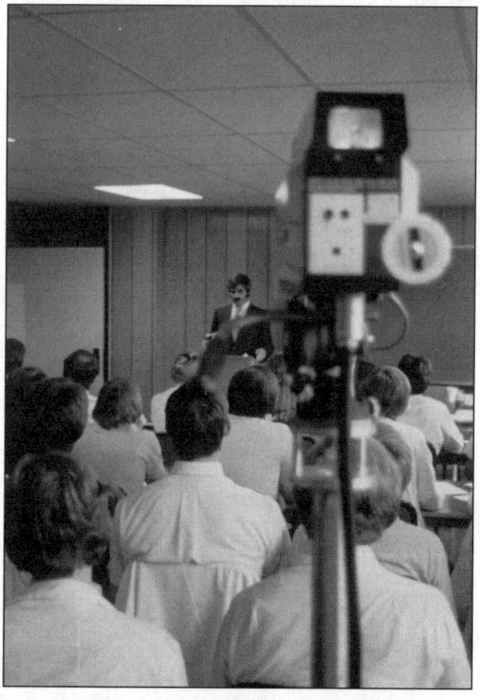

Revolutionary Med Wave technology connected students between hospital and classroom in the 1970s.

There were homes where the Roberts Research Center was later built, and in one of them lived a man nicknamed Mohammed. He walked up and down Ninth Street wearing African dress, carrying a staff, and preaching loudly. Eventually the school reached out more to that larger community, as for example with its extensive mentoring program in cooperation with Park School. But in the early 1980s, it was focused on the

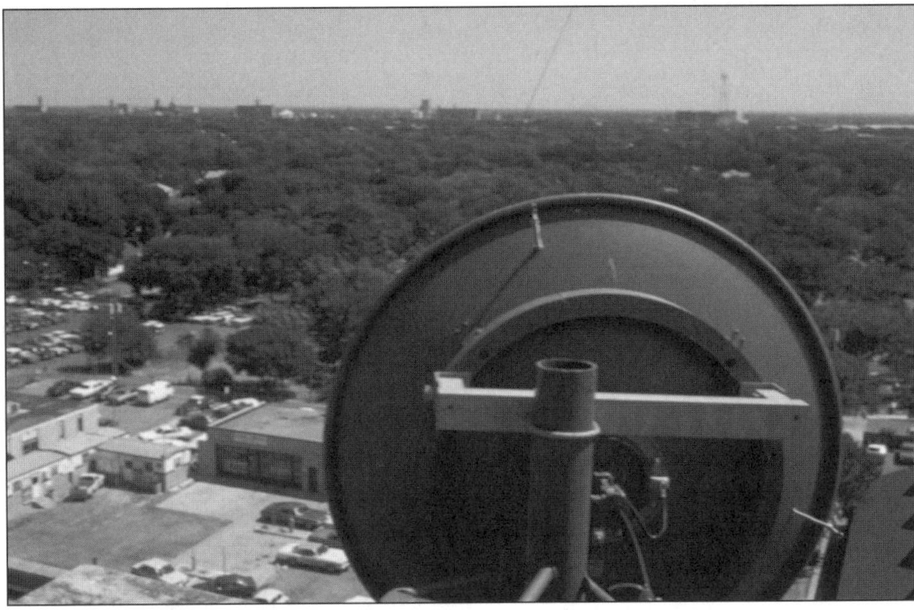

The Med Wave dish atop Wesley facing Via Christi-St. Francis.

mission to "find its own place," and to establish an identity. The last inpatients from Sedgwick County moved out of the building in 1981. About the same time a traffic sign went up on Highway I-135 identifying the KUSM-W exit, Dr. Voth commented, "We are not the branch."[419]

Certainly, the philosophy of the place had not changed with the changes in its physical plant. Dr. Dan Roberts, for instance, continued to be outspoken about the advantages of the community-based education system. Until recently, he wrote in 1979, childbirth had been a big killer of women. And improvements in that were not all due to things that could be learned in textbooks. "The students must develop an understanding for women and the very personal nature of the problems with which this specialty deals." Roberts had been though "the arrogant era" where physicians told patients what to do and had also been through an era "with women who assert themselves." One had to respond to some people one way and to others quite differently, and that was as much art and humanities as it was science. "If students can develop sensitivity to patients as individuals they will have accomplished much more than the act of treatment, they will understand the art of healing."[420]

People came and went. Dean Kortge was one who left. He was thirty-five, and from a perspective of later years thought that explained partly why he was resentful about the loss of Reed. He thought, too, that the spirit of the place would change, and that, should he stay, his role, experimental as it was, would change more than most. He had family in

Oregon and he was drawn there. But he thought leaving was the right thing. "KU was definitely going to put their imprimatur on the branch."[421]

Others continued the association, but agreed with Kortge that the atmosphere was changing, probably had to change as the institution matured. But they missed the old days in some ways. Dr. Lauren Welch, a neurologist, had a considerable literary and theological background for a physician, as well as being more of a free thinker than minimal independence might require. He observed there was a "collusion of anonymity" in the academic world, where it seemed sometimes that no individual was directly responsible for things. He thought that KUSM-W in the 1980s was becoming more like the regular academic world. Welch had a strong bias in favor of direct relationship and against teams, committees, and hierarchies, and therefore, while proud to see the school "growing up," realized that there are things all too "adult" about adults.[422]

Dr. R. Lawrence Sifford noted of this period that the trends in the 1980s at KUSM-W were nothing other than "classic institutionalization" and was a "very routine" development. The practitioners, he thought, were not courted so much as before. There was "nothing nasty" about that, he thought, just the idea that "we have our institution and we will run it and we are doing fine. I got the feeling that the practitioners shrugged and felt the same way." But all recognized that medicine was a "human experience and very complex," so some people felt, as Sifford did, that it was "kind of sad but very inevitable" that the institution of KUSM-W became more of an institution, and that the tensions with KUMC abated partly because KUSM-W became more like the mother institution.

In 1980, Dr. Walsh resigned as dean of KUSM-W, giving as an official reason that he wanted to get back to the Southwest.[423] He later recalled that his major mission from Chancellor Dykes had been to calm the town-gown tension in Wichita, and that he felt his speech to the Medical Society of Sedgwick County had done much to accomplish that. Dykes resigned his position at the University of Kansas just a few months after the departure of Walsh and went into private business, perhaps making it desirable again to have a long-time Wichitan at the helm in Wichita.[424] Walsh's replacement was just such a man, Dr. William Reals.

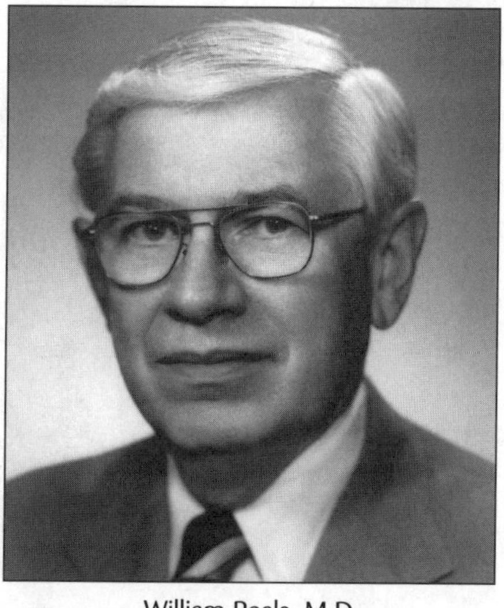

William Reals, M.D.

Although there was a contrast between the way Walsh had operated the place and the style of Reed, there was no doubt that Walsh had been mentored by Reed and had come to Wichita partly because of his achievements in outreach and rural medicine in New Mexico and the mesh of those concerns with Reed's sense of KUSM-W's mission. Reals had the long-standing local connections that Walsh had lacked, but he was, with his military background, more of an organization man who understood hierarchy and teamwork very well. Walsh felt that he got on well in the bureaucracy, but his former and later career suggest he was not wholly comfortable with it.

After leaving Wichita, Walsh became first Director of Emergency Medicine at the University of New Mexico School of Medicine, then was associated with the Indian Health Service in Phoenix, Arizona, and eventually directed the emergency medical program in Phoenix.[425] In 1988, he wrote an article for *Medical Economics* entitled "The Right Moves Nearly Killed Me." He said that at age sixty-two he could recognize that through his fast track life he had been "playing a role." He was, he said, "so wrapped up in being a physician that I forgot there was more to life." He developed ulcers at age forty-four, at which time he was involved in a half-dozen sideline businesses including an auto dealership. His first move out of the stressful life was to give up his practice "for a modest university salary." The second was his second marriage in 1980. In 1988, he enjoyed hiking and bicycling. He had no sideline businesses, no life insurance, and professed that his later life was a better life. That sense that there was much more to life than medicine Walsh had in common with Reed, and not too much in common with a good number of physicians, academic and clinical. So his departure from KUSM-W reinforced a change of mood.

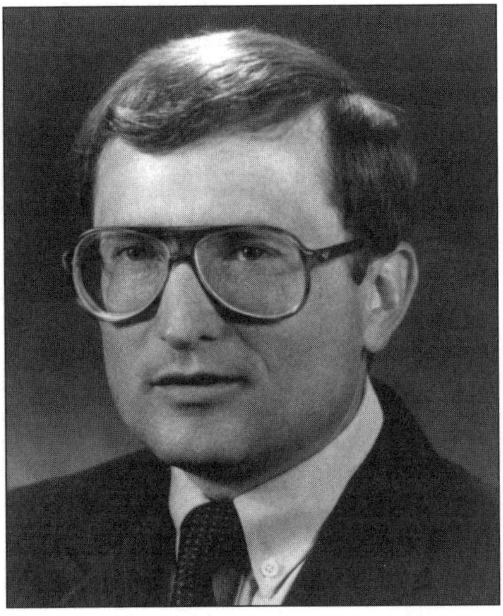

Gene Budig, M.D.

At the same time there was a change at the top at the University of Kansas. Dr. Gene Budig, forty-one years old, replaced Dykes as KU chancellor in 1981, and remained in that position until 1994.[426] Budig was a relatively young man, had no baggage concerning past administrative decisions and quickly got a strong feeling for the importance of KUSM-W to the University of Kansas. KUSM-W, Budig said, "gave the institution a very close partnership with the community. It became a very, very important component for the University of Kansas Medical Center." It opened doors for KU with physicians in Wichita and, Budig thought, "clearly operated in the best interests of the state. What's more, Wichita was popular with KU medical students. They had "excellent experiences" there and the faculty at Wichita was "especially responsive to student needs." Reals was in place when Budig arrived, but the new chancellor was happy with that choice. Reals knew the Wichita community and, in Budig's words, "went to great lengths to explain the school and what it would mean to the future of the region and the state." He wore well in the community and was "believable" on both campuses. Any lingering idea that Wichita was "Siberia," or a second rate "stepchild," Budig tried to root out at Lawrence and Kansas City. He thought that with each passing year there was greater appreciation at KUMC for the "potential and contribution" of KUSM-W. The cross-fertilization between academic and practice, Budig thought, was ideal, and "worked for both sides." Students at Wichita felt "they had been well prepared to practice medicine in a Midwestern setting." They liked the school and the city. Budig cultivated KU graduates in Wichita, such as Jordan Haines and Don Slawson, both of whom were members of the Board of Regents. He used the airplanes owned by KU more than chancellors before him to link the geographically separate parts of the single KU system. This involved spending several days a month in Wichita. He found there was no substitute for regular face-to-face contact with the people who made up the institution's component parts.

Budig did not see a crisis. "The initial objectives were the right ones," he said, and the early leaders had "built a solid foundation." It just took time for any institution to earn "real understanding and appreciation." By the time Budig left office in 1994 he felt there had been "enormous progress" in that area, and that KUSM-W had by then "widespread acceptance in Wichita and the rest of the state." No one in Kansas City by then seriously questioned the need for it.

Budig told his successor, Dr. Robert Hemenway, that the Wichita community took enormous pride in KUSM-W and that it was important that any KU chancellor early on "gain complete understanding of it." He told Hemenway, "It was deemed by many to be a central component of the total health science picture in Kansas. It was not a junior partner, it was a central component."

Budig, however optimistic, was also a realist, of course. He knew that physicians tended to resent bureaucracy and relate uncomfortably

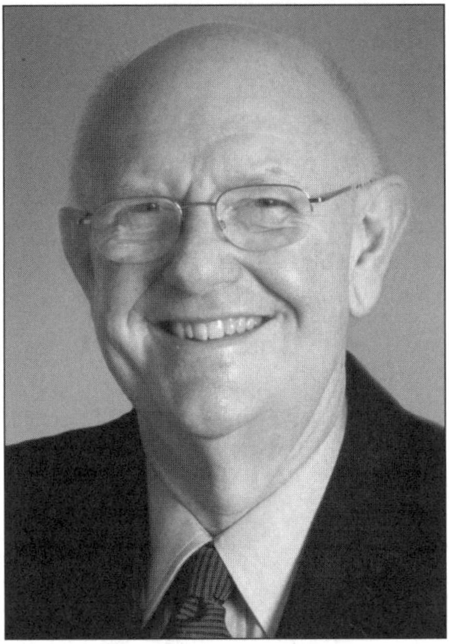

KU Chancellor Robert Hemenway

to institutions of any kind. One on one, he quipped later, medical doctors are very enjoyable "but as a group they can be difficult. They save lives; they have little time for trivia." There had to be a bureaucracy, but getting the faculty adjusted to it was done slowly and one detail at a time.[427]

Within the faculty, it was certainly far from all maverick resistance. Dr. Anne Walling started as a volunteer at KUSM-W just as Reals became dean and became a full-time faculty member in 1983. She had no connection with, and no particular nostalgia for, the pioneering days. Like many faculty who were part of the 1980s growth and change, she thought the new dispensation was very positive, particularly because there was less tension with Lawrence and Kansas City and more movement toward developing along consensus lines. Walling regarded Reals as the person "who made this place and gave it credibility." For one thing, he had "true academic credibility" as a pathologist and a national reputation in the forensics of aircraft accidents. And real credibility as a scientist was what was required in the leadership of an institution that wanted that same thing to rub off on it. It also required research, whatever the original idea of the legislature about the role of research in Wichita might have been.

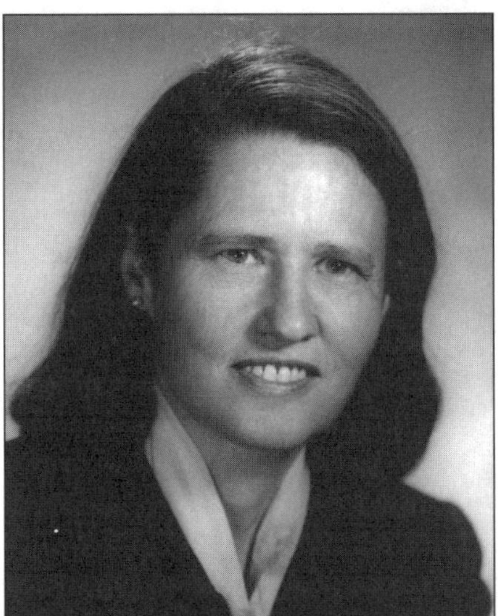

Anne Walling, M.B., Ch.B.

Reals got control of the situation in a "firm but gentle way," and, Walling thought, made the difference between success and failure.[428] Everyday examples remembered by staff included that when Reals instituted a no smoking policy he removed the ashtrays from the conference room. This caused Dr. Roberts to boycott the meetings for a time, and then to sit in the hall and yell out his comments. Reals simply let time pass, and eventually that storm blew over. RoxAnn Dicker, appointed by Reals as an associate dean despite her lack of a medical degree, believed that he added much to the formula. He held dean's meetings at eight o'clock in the morning with flags present in the conference room and portraits of the founders in the background. Things were more structured, Dicker remembered. Reals asked for a briefing, was good at gathering facts and "defined the institution and discipline."[429]

Walling also became an associate dean at KUSM-W, as did Jan Arbuckle. Arbuckle utilized the new computers to put the budget, accounting, payroll, and human resources on a more scientific basis than ever. She had been a budget analyst for the City of Wichita and had a degree in political science from WSU. She liked not only the organization and discipline typical of KUSM-W in the 1980s, but also the serious responsibilities she was given—opportunities that might not have been available in a larger or different organization. There was no facsimile machine, so all communications with KU went by mail, giving KUSM-W a bit of autonomy by default. It did inconvenience things that payroll warrants were still sent down the turnpike, and there was at least one occasion, before the advent of electronic bank deposits, when the highway patrol was called in to get them there on time. There was a "whole spectrum of different kinds of contractual obligations," concerning which the school had to develop policy. And there was the business end of things to apply to independent academics. A department chair once asked Arbuckle, "Why do I have to make my budget balance?" The answer was that this was no longer, if it ever was, a "mom and pop" operation, but big business. An "established decision-making bureaucracy" was needed, Arbuckle thought, however much people thought they could or should get along without one. Reals reigned in what Arbuckle called the "fireworks of personality," and integrated those personalities into a system. Deans, she philosophized, played a "critical role in cajoling and keeping the lions on their perches."

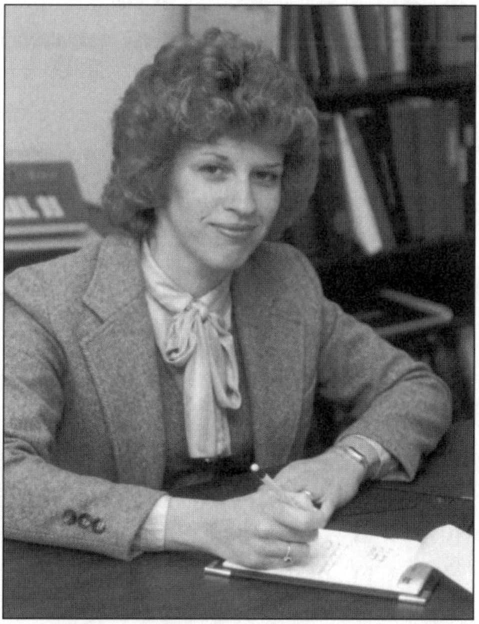
Jan Arbuckle, Associate Dean for Administration

The deans that followed could "capitalize on the civility the other deans created and can move us in new directions." KUSM-W was lucky in having deans with longevity, and that would not have happened had they not been "masters at relationship building."[430]

Walling much appreciated the greater stability and credibility she saw emerging at Wichita in the 1980s and 1990s. The school needed money and money did not come from rebels. Nor was the state legislature particularly interested in the innovative or experimental except on the fringes. Walling was tired of there always seeming to be an underlying question about Wichita, "Are you just private practitioners who take students into your office or are you really teachers?" It was time for an end to the nervous period—what she called the "sky is falling times." KUSM-W had a wonderful teaching paradigm, small class, a small faculty, and a "very clear vision of the end product." It needed to parlay that into a solid organizational future. In the mid-1980s, she thought, computers and credibility arrived at about the same time. Individual faculty had always had this credibility. Roberts, who used to have a Chicago policeman's nightstick across his desk, and Farha, Walling remembered, continued to be the "muscle" with Kansas City, Lawrence, and Topeka when that was needed. But the institution as institution lacked a strong image, and what image it had was blurred and not altogether favorable. When the light finally shined on a substantial school, it had to reveal the right things. In Walling's view, that was exactly what happened in the 1980s. Those were, she said, "very exciting times" at the school. They were times when people at KUSM-W "woke up to medical education" as an academic and "not just an osmotic process." Medical education, she concluded, had to be more than just a bunch of smart people hanging around together. For all the laughable features on the surface of the academic world, especially as seen by those at a distance, there were aspects at its core that were tremendously serious and vitally important to any medical school that planned to survive in the late twentieth century.[431]

Of all the women who prospered at KUSM-W, none had longer standing nor in many ways a more remarkable record than Lorene Valentine. She made the transition from Reed, to whom she had been perhaps closer than anyone else, with aplomb. She had known Reals since the 1960s, which helped. She became the Assistant Dean for Administration in the spring of 1981 and later Associate Dean, even though, as she put it, as a female without a master's degree at that time she might have seemed an unlikely candidate. But Reals shared Reed's penchant for "collecting people," rather than simply resumes. Valentine, who eventually worked for all the deans of KUSM-W, and who had watched all the political struggles of the 1970s, admired the skills of Reals within a bureaucratic structure. "Reals," she commented, "knew how to play that." What he may have lacked in charisma compared to Reed, he made up for in a strong pragmatic sense of what would work. Reed, by contrast, had been known to push a "non-starter" idea too far.[432]

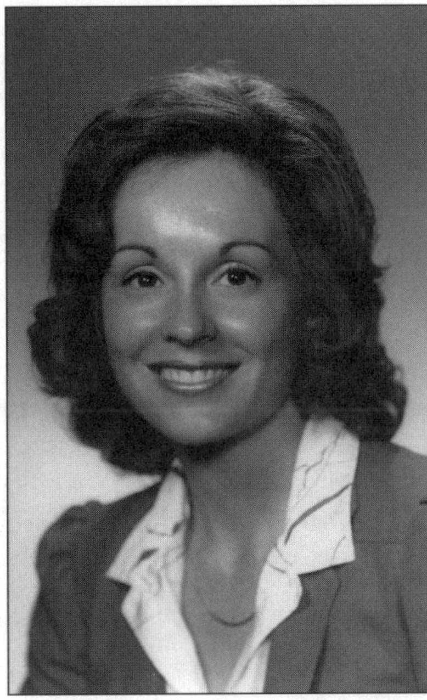

Lorene Valentine, the school's first Associate Dean for Administration

One might add thumbnail biographies of other faculty members to illustrate the changes further. Dr. Sechin Cho is a good example. He joined the medical school in the Department of Pediatrics in 1978, after finishing his residency and a fellowship at Johns Hopkins. Cho loved the "hands-on" aspects of medical education in Wichita. "We teach them where they are going to work," and when they get out, they are "doing the same thing in the same environment." But Cho was also a specialist in genetics, and there was hardly a more research-dependent, more equipment-intensive, or more fundamentally academic field. Recognizing that Wichita was not designed to have basic science in the

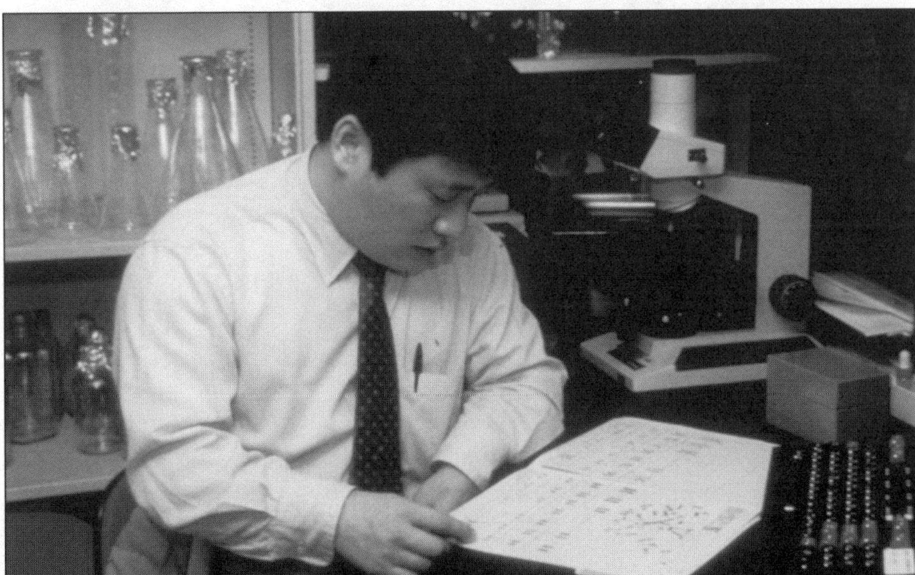

Sechin Cho, M.D.

curriculum, Cho thought it had to emphasize clinical research for faculty and he approved of the trend to do so. He, like many others, was glad to see any undercurrent of Wichita's having a competitive ambition for a full-blown medical school disappear. He was glad to see KUSM-W in the 1980s concentrate on training clinical physicians. That was the way to survive and prosper.[433]

"It was hard to work with KU when we were so small," Hazel Fenske recalled, "now we are all right. We proved ourselves."[434] KUSM-W became, Dr. Richard Shaw claimed, the "showplace in the country in how to run someplace like this."[435] Naturally myriad ground-level details affected the evolution of the place so that such statements were eventually believable. Strategic integration of these into a consistent mission was a tall order well met as the school's second decade passed. But fulfilling it would create the "best of both worlds" type of institution for which the Wichita faculty had hoped all along.

Chapter Eight

MATURE

When Dr. Cramer Reed was recognized late in 1980 by the naming of a lecture hall at the CHRP at WSU in his honor, he summed up what it took to build a "truly fine professional health school," and by implication a fine medical school. The main thing was understanding, "the mutual interdependence of the various parts comprising the system." He observed, "Too often we fail to appreciate the perspective, the viewpoint, and even the value of the various parts that comprise the whole. This lack of understanding makes difficult the development, the sense of common purpose, so necessary for success. Instead, it becomes easy to lapse into mistrust and cynicism about what others are thinking and doing."[436]

In some significant ways, what KUSM-W in the 1980s was doing was institutionalizing that sense of common purpose so as to spend more time advancing and less time distrusting the differences that could easily dominate.

It was not easy. Faculty morale had been mixed, with significant turnover among the full-time people. Dr. Glodys St. Phard left in 1979 to join the faculty at the College of Medicine of South Alabama with the statement to the press, "I cannot be part of what I perceive as an academic dead end." He thought the legislature was giving KUSM-W only enough support "to keep its head above water." Dr. Douglas Young commented at the same time, "How long can you be in a developmental stage?" Dr. Hewitt Goodpasture thought it looked suspiciously as though there was "nothing that had been invested by the state at Wichita since 1973 that could not be divested." When KUSM-W requested seventeen new faculty members for the 1980 budget, the regents reduced that to ten and the legislature cut it to two. The legislature was providing $40,000 salaries on average for full-time people and the rest had to be generated by the practice corporation. That organization, however, could not bridge the gap entirely in the finances that were needed for excellence.[437]

At the time, there remained an image problem. For instance, in the summer of 1980, the *Wichita Eagle* wrote that the school had an "extended identity crisis." That following February, the president of the Wichita Area Chamber of Commerce spoke to the Medical Society of Sedgwick County about health care in the 1980s and never even mentioned KUSM-W. Because people were usually unsupportive of things they did not understand, increasing understanding was vital. So in the fall of 1981, a consultant was hired to study the school for two months. He talked to officials, employees, physicians, members of the media, and townspeople. He reviewed newspaper clippings and read reports. His conclusion was, "without question, the school lacks visibility in the community." Still, things were improving. The Division of Health Care Outreach had received excellent press through the state, so much so that, the report concluded," it is likely that KUSM-W is better known in the rural areas of Kansas than in Wichita." The Mobile Continuing Education Program reached 4,000 rural health professionals a year. The Division of Postgraduate Education planned and implemented twenty major conferences a year. And then there were the new signs on the interstate.

There remained "a number of natural irritations," the report said, but these were decreasing. An active public relations program would aid further to advance the goal of "doing good and getting credit for it." It was a function of the school's administration "to evaluate public attitudes, identify the policies and programs with the public interest, and then plan and execute a program of action to earn public understanding and acceptance." The public relations program "would be a determined effort to motivate or influence people—primarily through communication—to think well of the school, to respect it, to support it, and to stick with it through trial and trouble. It is important to build up a bank account of credibility through good works." Every letter dispatched from KUSM-W, the consultant said, "should be written with thought to its possible influence on prestige and goodwill." The publications and the speaker's bureau should all be coordinated, and perhaps the publications changed in type and makeup. Quality was vital, not only in the advertising, but in the product. "A good medical school can be held in less than high regard by the public because of poor public relations, but a mediocre medical school cannot expect to cover up its shortcomings with an aggressive public relations program. Good relations come about when a medical school fulfills its purpose . . . and then proceeds to interpret this to its various publics. When this is done, public understanding will come—slowly but certainly."[438]

But all saw there was excellence anyway. Dr. Cho was one of only four geneticists in the state. He used amniocentesis and sonograms among other things to provide genetic counseling to at risk patients at the neonatal center at Wesley hospital, and was supported by the National Foundation/March of Dimes.[439] Dr. E.P. Donatelle, who came from the University of North Dakota in 1979 to become chair of the Department of Family Practice in Wichita, was the editor of a renowned textbook entitled *Family Medicine: Principles and Practice*.[440] Dr. Richard Guthrie in the early 1980s was pioneering in the care of diabetes. Wichita became nationally known through the work of Guthrie and his wife Diana, who was an R.N., in the use of increasingly smaller computers for the automatic and constant regulation of blood sugar and in some of the first tests of synthetic insulin in the nation. The two also wrote numerous books on the topic. In fact, he became so much involved in this, and with diabetes patient care through the KUSM-W Practice Association, that he moved away from a strict pediatric specialty and from the full-time academic work he was doing when first hired.[441] Dr. Ernest Crow was all too modest at his retirement in 1988 in saying that he had only shared in the "golden age of cardiology. It's gone from a field where you can do virtually nothing to a field where you can do a lot."[442] Crow did much pioneering in bringing heart procedures to the city. "Our abilities to precisely define a problem are pretty good," he commented. "And our abilities to fix a problem are pretty good. So many of us are thinking that the next breakthrough will be some medical treatment for heart disease."[443] Apropos of that and an appropriate honor for KUSM-W's first department chair for internal medicine, in 1989, KUSM-W, with a $100,000 grant from the Claude R. Lambe Charitable Foundation established a cardiac lab to study rhythm abnormalities. The facility would, said the dean, "give physicians a better chance of pinpointing discrete areas in the heart responsible for rhythm abnormalities. Since

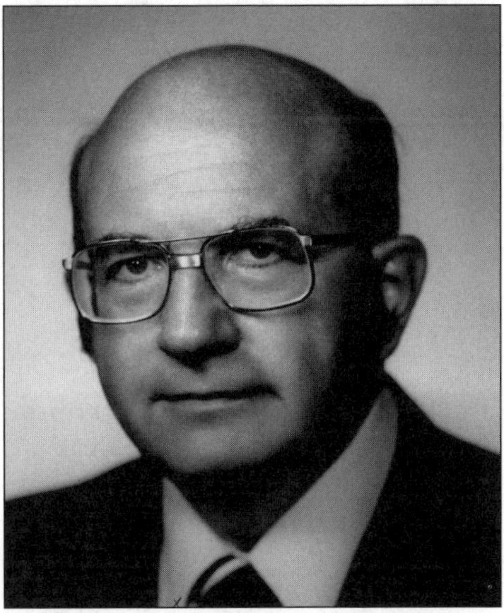

E.P Donatelle, M.D.

rhythm disorders are still among the most difficult and complex problems in cardiology, it is a fertile field for research."[444]

Roberts continued to be "whirling dervish of achievement." Always, he was outgoing and enthusiastic and quotable. He hugged male friends and cried at movies. He told the local paper in 1981, when being interviewed on his fortieth birthday, "There's not much about medicine that I don't like."[445]

The Women's Research Institute and its applied arm, the Center for Reproductive Medicine, founded in 1984 as joint ventures of Wesley Medical Center and KUSM-W, were in many ways Roberts's most impressive monuments. In 1978, Louise Brown of Great Britain became the world's first "test tube baby," conceived in a laboratory setting and transferred to the womb. That so few years later, one of the most advanced and statistically successful clinics and research operations in male and female infertility should be located in a two-story former church in Wichita, Kansas, was a tribute to Roberts's scientific enthusiasm and entrepreneurial drive. Dr. Bobby Webster, whose picture, along with Roberts's, adorned the center's elegant and modern headquarters attached to the refurbished KUSM-W headquarters at the former E.B. Allen, was in charge of the day-to-day operation of the Center for Reproductive Medicine. Dr. Brooks Keel, a specialist in male infertility, joined him in 1985. These men were serious researchers as well as ultra-specialists and strengthened KUSM-W's staff as well as their own business.[446] It was leading edge from the first, having in 1986, for example, one of three computerized sperm analysis machines in the U.S.[447] The first Wichita birth of a baby conceived by *in vitro* fertilization took place in the summer of 1988.[448] Keel commented, "Infertility, just because it doesn't kill you, does not make it any less serious than a tumor. It's a disease."[449] It might have been a frustration to the doctors at the center that they probably got more local publicity for removing eggs from a dying orangutan at the Sedgwick County Zoo than from their work with people but, as with KUSM-W itself, awareness and appreciation of the core mission in the community was slow and took years of accomplishment to establish.[450]

The sale of Wesley Medical Center in 1985 for over $200 million created a wealthy foundation dedicated to advancing health care in the region. Clearly, that was an opportunity for KUSM-W, particularly in the area of expanding what had been one of its weak spots, research. It also boded well, according to its proponents, for improving hospital care in a high technology, high capital expense era. Roberts thought the sale was for both reasons "an act of extraordinary foresight," in that it allowed the resources of a hospital chain to be applied to the needs of an individual

Wichita hospital, and would create a fund for the support of medical education.[451] Certainly, it had an enormous effect. By 2004, the Wesley Foundation and its successor, the Kansas Health Foundation, had granted over $46 million to KUMC and KUSM-W.[452]

There was a tremendous run by the Wesley Foundation (assets $250 million) and its president Duane Dyer in the mid-1980s to establish a nationally important biomedical research institute in Wichita, a project in which KUSM-W and its faculty were intimately involved. By 1987, the foundation had made 175 grants and fellowships totaling over $1.2 million, focused increasingly on medical education and research. Ironically in some ways, this project began to re-establish the connection between KUSM-W and Wichita State University so painfully broken in 1978. For a proposal to advance "bench" or basic research, the existing resources of the university in basic science, intellectual and physical, were vital.[453]

It certainly excited the community. Health care, wrote a reporter in 1987, could put the city in the national spotlight. It was an area where Wichita already had a "significant presence," and with the addition of Wesley Foundation funding for research, health care could become an industry cluster of the status of aviation for Wichita. It was a question of achieving take-off momentum in the industry and of what kind of money and innovation that would require. Warren Oblinger, a city planner, spoke of a "health care corridor" that ran from the river east on Murdock past the St. Francis Hospital campus, KUSM-W and the Sedgwick County Department of Health to Hillside, then north along Hillside to WSU and south to Wesley Medical Center, the Wichita Clinic, and St. Joseph Hospital. Could Wichita not become "a research, development, training, production, warehousing, distribution, and administrative center for health care related business and industry?"[454]

WSU in 1987 prepared a grant proposal to the Wesley Foundation for a multi-million dollar center. Averett Tombes, vice president for research and graduate studies at WSU, said that he wanted the facility to tie together schools, hospitals, and businesses interested in biomedical research. "I'm taking a leadership role for the biomedical community already in Wichita." Dr. Reals at KUSM-W chimed in with support, noting that KUSM-W had cooperated with WSU before.[455] One spokesperson for the Chamber of Commerce envisioned "Wichita as a national powerhouse in health care, fueled by cooperation between the city's major hospitals and educational facilities. This vision releases Wichita workers from the stranglehold of a fluctuating aircraft economy, while at the same time mapping out a future in which Wichita can grow and prosper."[456] KUSM-W in 1987 mounted a public relations campaign with the slogan: "KUSM-W and Wichita—Good for Each Other."[457]

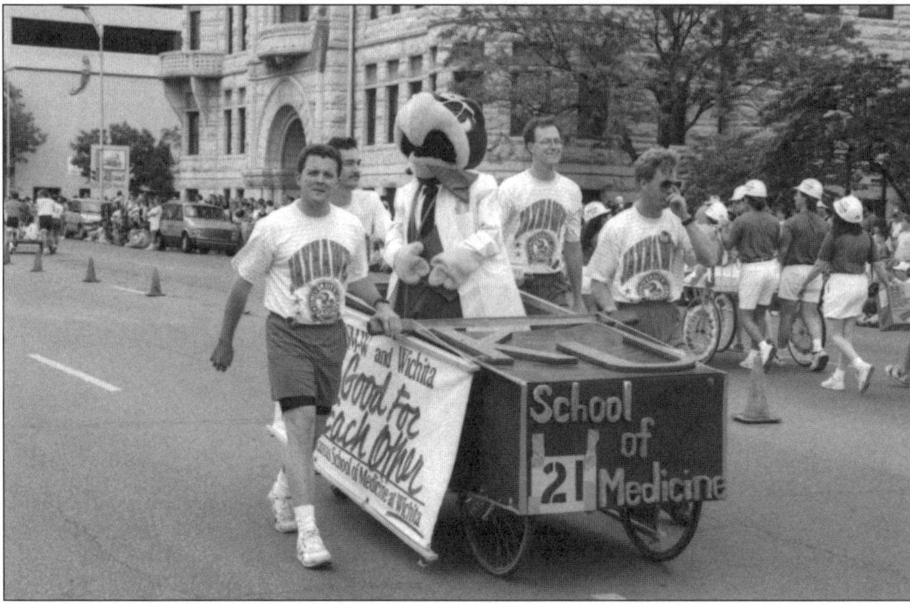

In the 1980s, KUSM-W began to take an active part in community activities.

The biomedical research center concept never came to fruition.[458] The task of creating enough of a basic research complex in Wichita to attract top people, and of getting the whole thing moving, originally was beyond even the resources of the Wesley Foundation. However, it was a strong try, and a move in a promising direction at the beginning of the human genome project. Clearly many industries in the future would compete for and employ "knowledge workers," and market "software" ideas and solutions more than foundry castings. And KUSM-W and others in Wichita had that trend right in the mid-1980s. The school had the opportunity then to expand exponentially, not only in physical size, but also in the scope of its mission, and it did try to attach itself to a train that unfortunately never left the station. The newspaper noted that it was a "Catch-22" situation: the Center for Molecular Medicine "is unable to build the critical mass without a director who can attract other scientists and research dollars, but it is unable to attract a director without much of the critical mass in place."[459] Still, there was excitement in being involved in leading edge achievement. Dr. James Farha, who with his brother George, the department chair of surgery at KUSM-W, ran a very successful surgery practice and had done 2,000 coronary artery bypasses since the team pioneered them in Wichita in 1968, told a reporter, "What can you do that's more challenging? It's not taking out ingrown toenails."[460]

As vital as the new directions were, however, there was no abandonment of some of the older features that had given KUSM-W its special character from the outset. Primary among these, perhaps, was outreach. It reached out to the Wichita community from its own site and cooperated with other local organizations in improving medical care for the city to all groups and on all levels. Dr. Sue Menking, a pediatrician working with KUSM-W, and others established a clinic for the Mid-America All-Indian Center in Wichita. There were 3,800 Indians in Wichita, and the clinic was one of forty-one urban health programs in the U.S. for Native Americans funded by federal grants.[461] By 1982, there were several outpatient clinics operating at KUSM-W, including one on birth defects. Classrooms at four Wichita hospitals were linked to the school by two-way closed circuit television.[462] In 1984, the Department of Psychiatry established an outpatient clinic for the treatment and evaluation of the violent—people subject to unpredictable and uncontrollable outbursts of rage. Co-directed by Dr. Neil Roach and Dr. Glenn Vennstra of KUSM-W, it used multi-disciplinary techniques and was the only program of its kind in Kansas.[463] Roach had found that there were few entrepreneurial psychiatric activities in town. Most of the people were trained at the Menninger Clinic in Topeka and had an analytic and Freudian-based background, as contrasted with biochemical and eclectic approaches. Roach commented that it was "narcissistic to think that the sound of your voice will cure illness." In addition to the focus on treating violent personalities, Roach and associates had a good deal of success with eating disorders.[464] On a less grandiose level, perhaps, but serving a useful purpose was Dr. Anne Walling's *ex cathedra* advice to the local papers on the treatment of chigger bites, certainly a perennial Kansas problem.[465]

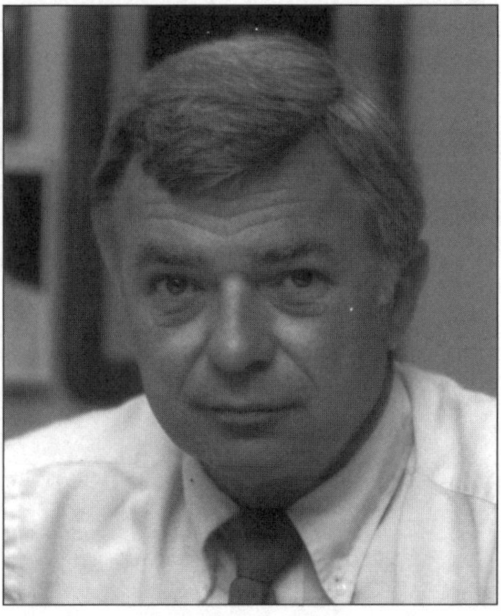

Neil Roach, M.D.

Working with other Wichita institutions became a near art. In 1982, KUSM-W helped develop a short care children's program housed at St. Joseph Hospital. The Department of Psychiatry at KUSM-W emphasized the need for this program, noting that there had been attempts at suicide in children as young as six, and that problems like school phobia, resulting in sickness in the morning, were common. This program would provide short-term diagnostic evaluation and recommendations.[466] Another cooperative program with large potential social effect was a teen clinic, which began operation in a small yellow aluminum-sided house near North High School in 1988. One in sixteen high school seniors drank daily. Six percent of the boys and 15 percent of the girls had been sexually abused. Half of the city's rape victims were under age eighteen. Five thousand children under age nineteen committed suicide in the U.S. Ten percent of girls had severe eating disorders. Teenagers committed one-third of violent crimes, and yet they utilized health care services less than any other segment of the population. However controversial the teen clinic was (and its distribution of contraceptives made it controversial), three members of the Department of Pediatrics at KUSM-W participated in the clinic, which was funded on a year-to-year basis by the state legislature. Dr. Gerard VanLeeuwen, professor and chair of the department, was interviewed often by the local media, and it gave him a chance to outline the magnitude of the problems which this little clinic tried to address.[467] The same year, and to much more acclaim, KUSM-W's Department of Family and Community Medicine offered a weight loss class in Wichita, twelve weeks for $150. Participants had to be 25 percent over their optimum weight. Dr. Beth Alexander, who oversaw it, said it had the benefit of raising self-esteem as well as improving physical health. "We don't just say a person is overweight," she commented, "we say they're ugly or lazy or sinful or stupid." Through role-playing, behavior modification, and better nutrition, the program hoped to change all that.[468]

Important also were lecture series and workshops in Wichita, many co-sponsored with other local educational and medical institutions. Whether it was a program on medical malpractice pitting Dr. Roberts against Kathleen Sebelius of the Trial Lawyers Association, or a Senior Wellness Education and Testing program, or a lecture in the Francis Schiltz series sponsored by KUSM-W, or a speech by Dr. Beth Alexander on "Talking with Kids About Sensitive Subjects," or a seminar on hyperactivity in children and the relative effectiveness of Ritalin and the popular Feingold Diet, there was constant opportunity for Wichitans to learn more about medicine through the efforts of the school.[469] KUSM-W was a co-sponsor of an annual International Conference on Human Functioning with the Center for the Improvement of Human Functioning, an alternative medicine center focused on diet and nutrition.[470]

Nor was institutional jealousy a factor. Kansas State University (KSU) had a dietetics program that required seniors there to spend one semester at the KSU Dietetics Center in Wichita working with doctors and community agencies. Beginning in the fall of 1987, these students worked also with third and fourth year medical students at KUSM-W. The head of KSU's hotel restaurant, institutional management and dietetics program much appreciated that. "Even though our students were in the hospitals every day, making rounds with doctors and medical students," she said, "they were completely isolated." Dr. Joseph Meek, who had moved to Wichita from Kansas City to become chair of the Department of Internal Medicine at KUSM-W, was instrumental in aiding this cooperation by not only encouraging interchange, but offering offices to two KSU faculty at E.B. Allen and allowing KSU students to use Medline at KUSM-W. The KSU people exclaimed, "there is nothing that's close to us here." Meek commented that it was only enlightened self-interest by KUSM-W. "In the past teaching patients about nutrition meant giving them a pamphlet and a printed diet." Now the experts were on the scene.[471]

Perhaps the most exciting outreach, however, was the remote outreach, particularly in providing education and services to western Kansas, an area long considered to be Wichita's natural trading territory and perhaps, in the modern age, also its natural medium for information exchange. Health Day continued, drawing about 100 students for a lunch meeting in 1981 to meet with representatives from small towns.[472] By the 1980s, about 80 percent of students at KUSM and KUSM-W took advantage of a tuition forgiveness program that required them to spend some time in a medically underserved area of Kansas in order to receive their education at a reduced rate.[473] The real goal, however, was that more doctors remain in these areas for their entire careers. Dean Waxman of KUMC spent time in 1985 observing Dr. Rick Kellerman, preparing for a career in family practice, working at Plainville, north of Hays. Plainville was one of eleven communities selected by KUSM-W as a place to establish preceptorships. Students spent part of their time working with doctors in small towns, and thus learning well in advance of their own decisions about where to locate their own practices and what the advantages and disadvantages of such situations were. A good part of the stereotypes overcome were negative ones and, on the whole, the experiences resulted in a more positive view by students of the possibilities of small town practice.[474] Seniors served these preceptorships in non-urban areas, it was said, to "further their awareness of professional opportunities in primary care."[475] Some town programs were more elaborate than simply preceptorships. There had been a significant program at Harper in the 1970s, and in 1980, with the cooperation of KUSM-W, Salina established a family practice clinic where eight resident physicians would spend two years training as family practice specialists. They would see their own patients and be assigned to local doctors on a rotating basis. This had been in planning at Wichita since 1976, and funding came from a three-year federal grant.[476]

Simple preceptorships, however, were the bread and butter of the outreach program. David Bollig chose WaKeeney in 1985 for his preceptorship, and extended his rural family practice experience with Dr. James Hamilton there from four weeks to four months. Bollig happened to be from nearby Plainville himself, and his experience indicated how closely related recruiting for the classes was to eventual placement. People from the area did not need any orientation to western Kansas culture.[477] Faculty reached out to the area, also. Dr. Dennis Finley, a clinical assistant professor of surgery at KUSM-W, and a specialist in reconstructive surgery on the hand and foot, was in Russell, Kansas, on Wednesdays. Other specialists would appear on other days.[478] Dr. Guthrie held diabetes seminars in Russell in 1985, too, to complete the cross section of care.[479] Seminars such as the one titled "The Right to Live and the Right To Die," held for doctors, nurses, and allied health professionals at the Edwards County Hospital in Kinsley in 1981 were typical of KUSM-W activity in formal outreach education.[480] That year, health care professionals from Hodgeman, Comanche, Edwards, Ford, Kiowa, Ness, Pawnee, Rush, and Stafford Counties heard numerous addresses on medical topics at the Edwards County location.[481] A fetal monitoring course was given the next year at Liberal in far southwestern Kansas. It was sponsored by KUSM-W, the perinatal program at Wesley Hospital, and the Southwest Medical Center at Liberal. It carried a three-hour credit toward relicensure.[482] Not everyone at KUSM-W went to the same trouble as Dr. Bruce Woods, a Wichita family therapist and clinical assistant professor, who in 1986 rode from town to town on a bicycle through eleven counties promoting a family wellness program.[483] But enthusiasm for being proactive at getting the word out was high.

Of course, at the core of things, were students and the student experience, and in that area, by all measures, KUSM-W was quite successful. Dr. Nancy Nowlin and Dr. Douglas Voth wrote an article in 1979 for the *Journal* of the Kansas Medical Society called "Basic Clerkship: Students in Internal Medicine on a Community Clinical Campus." It provided a succinct description of the basic student program in one department upon which the school was building, as well as reflecting a bit on the brief history of student life in Wichita.

When the first class of fourteen came in 1974, the clerkship in internal medicine lasted ten weeks. By 1979, the internal medicine clerkship was twelve weeks and the class was fifty. One full-time faculty member scheduled and coordinated the various activities of the clerkship. Others staffed teaching services and made teaching rounds with the students at all four major hospitals. Full-time, part-time, and volunteer faculty served as "primary attending physicians," to provide, each week, three new patients suitable for assignment to the students. This group reviewed the students' work and made teaching rounds three to five times per week. Certain "highly capable" part-time and volunteer faculty "who have exceptional patience and teaching skills" were asked to give short remedial courses for students who needed special academic support. During their clerkship weeks the students interviewed and examined thirty-six to forty patients.

The emphasis was on "problem identification and solving" rather than memorization of facts. Still, fact had to be mastered. "Although the clerkship is distinctly patient-oriented, formal, didactic-tutorial sessions are given twice weekly." These consisted of a thirty-minute faculty presentation and fifteen minutes of discussion. Some presentations dealt with common patient problems, such as headache. Others covered specific diseases, and still others were devoted to teaching a skill, such as the interpretation of electrocardiograms. Faculty reviewed student papers, conducted oral exams at the end of each clerkship, and presented and attended noon conferences and grand rounds.

The weekly schedule of a student was full. Primary attending physicians made bedside rounds three to five times a week in which students participated. "Professor Rounds" were conducted two days a week. These were formal presentations by a student and demonstration of findings followed by group discussion. Coordination of these was rotated among a few faculty members "who are selected for their special aptitudes and abilities to support, stimulate, lead, and evaluate the students in this kind of setting." There were clinical pathology rounds once a week, done jointly by a member of the full-time faculty of the Department of Internal Medicine and a faculty pathologist assigned by the KUSM-W Department of Pathology. In this, one or two patients were presented followed by a conference to review "clinicopathological correlations." Pertinent biopsy specimens on microscopic slides were utilized. All students taking the junior medical clerkship met at the medical school three times a week. Two meetings were for didactic tutorials. The third was with a full-time faculty member who coordinated the clerkship, and with the chairman. During this program, a student presented a patient and the group constructed a problem list and differential diagnoses and discussed the approach to the patient's problem. An effort was made to present patients with common complaints. Each student was required to write six critical case summaries during the twelve weeks of the clerkship. Papers were reviewed and critiqued by the attending physician and resident responsible for the patient as well as an independent outside faculty reviewer not involved in caring for the patient. Each hospital had a separate schedule of educational conferences in internal medicine, twelve to fifteen a week, throughout the city. Students were expected to attend these scholarly presentations by a faculty member or a visiting professor. The student's overall progress was discussed and reviewed in detail at faculty meetings every two weeks. There were written evaluations each six weeks. Topics for oral examinations were taken from a list of eight topics chosen by the student. Out of 1,000 possible points, 500 were from clinical and interpersonal skills, 200 from critical case summaries, 200 from the written exam, and 200 from an oral exam. The student had to score at least 700.

The whole clerkship, Voth and Nowlin thought, was more than the sum of its parts. "Working with community physicians, students are involved in the care of patients who are clearly representative of the population in this region. Most patients have common problems that are seen by internists, while many others are referred to our faculty in the tertiary care centers in this city because of esoteric or complicated conditions. All students have the opportunity to observe their faculty accept the risks, challenges, and rewards of caring for their own patients on a daily basis." The early "administrative obligation" to "integrate the various hospital components and resident and student education," was by 1980, the report thought, "largely accomplished."[484]

Certainly enrollments met all expectations. By the late 1980s, enrollment was averaging about 175. Women were about 30 percent (50 percent by the turn of the twenty-first century) and minorities represented about 11 percent of the class.[485]

Kansas City students chose Wichita willingly, eagerly. "I think they designed things more toward students' needs and for their education than Kansas City," said a consultant in 1989. Dr. Reals added, "Doctors in this town are anxious to teach the students." Classes were smaller than in Kansas City. Faculty-to-student ratio by the late 1980s was one faculty for every two students, as contrasted with one for every seven in Kansas City. Students were welcomed at the meetings of the Medical Society of Sedgwick County, and experience in Wichita might accustom students to a more western milieu. But mostly students just liked it. Said Kevin Rieg, a student, "They really treat you nicely down here. You are respected when you are working in the hospital. The staff bends over backwards for you. . . . The faculty is very interested in the students and they want the students to do well and they invest a personal interest in them. They, and the residency programs, have become known and have sent students to a big number of programs."[486] Said another student, "It's like heaven. There's a lot of individual attention."[487]

There was a sense in the middle and late 1980s that KUSM-W was a mature institution. It was hosting art exhibits.[488] The residencies at the hospitals, so long a kind of bone of contention across the town, merged in 1988 under the aegis of KUSM-W. The reason, Reals announced, was "to try to cut costs and strengthen academic standing." But it was also the result of a long, slow campaign by KUSM-W to gain credibility itself and to convince the hospitals to give up their traditional independent residency graduate programs.[489] The hospitals were locked in competition to become Level I trauma centers and to acquire the latest technology, so in many ways this result was a relief to them as well as a boon to KUSM-W.[490]

Dr. Reals and Jan Arbuckle, the associate dean for administration, authored a ten-year review of the school in 1984. It appeared in the Kansas Medical Society journal, and had an upbeat tone. State appropriations for KUSM-W had grown from $250,000 to more than $8 million a year during the period. Contractual revenue through the practice association reached $1.3 million in 1984. There was a complete medical illustration service, an inter-hospital color television microwave system for closed circuit communication, and a medical library. The Division of Postgraduate Education provided 100 programs to 3,000 people in 1983. The hypertension screening program had served 175,000 Kansans since 1974. Now called REACH (Respond Early and Control Hypertension) it was specializing in working with churches in the black community where uncontrolled hypertension was a particular problem. Medical school personnel, in conjunction with the Wichita Heart Association, worked with city and county fire stations in providing blood pressure measurement and follow-up service. The Senior Health Program reached 2,000 since 1981. The junior class was more than 50 percent female, compared with 30 percent in medical schools nationally. More than 3,500 physicians and 3,000 nurses each year attended the continuing education seminars sponsored by KUSM-W. A new patient care clinic opened at the school headquarters in 1983 and was serving seventy-five outpatients a day. Of the $12 million annual budget, $1.6 million went to area hospitals for financial support for students. "The School has made a major impact in health education as well as research," the review stated. "Because we are a medical school without walls, we depend upon the community of Wichita, the health professionals and the hospitals to work with us in our teaching program. The School is a prospering example of a community-based medical school, and we are proud of our accomplishments."[491]

In 1986, Dr. Cramer Reed "retired," insofar as he ever could, this time from his post as senior vice president at Wesley Medical Center. He still backpacked, river rafted, jogged, mountain climbed, and played handball three times a week. There couldn't be a better example of continuing good health.[492]

Dr. Daniel Roberts, a second icon of the early history of the school, was less lucky in health and vigorous age. He died at age fifty-seven on June 23, 1994. There was hardly room in any publication to list his many achievements in fields from electron microscopy to reproductive endocrinology to lobbying on medical malpractice changes. But surely prominent among those achievements was being part of the initial core of department chairs at KUSM-W. He had lived to see the Roberts Amphitheater opened at KUSM-W, and that was only the beginning of the continued associations with, and reflections of his life and career, as were built into that institution.[493] It seemed that the institution was thriving beyond the active careers and even the lives of the first generation of its promoters, which gave it a "tradition," if not exactly an ancient one.

There was even real recognition in Lawrence that KUSM-W had arrived as a permanent part of the state's medical education establishment. In the summer of 1989, the *Lawrence Journal World* ran a piece called "KU's 'other' Medical Center." KUSM-W was more than its modest administrative center, the reporter noted. "The heart of the program comes from the willing cooperation of four Wichita medical centers and hundreds of local physicians. Over 600 had graduated and of those 57 percent had chosen primary care specialties. Of 301 who had completed residency training, 165, or 55 percent, were practicing in Kansas. Dr. Joseph Meek, who had come to Wichita from a post at KUMC and knew the Kansas City organization well, commented, "We are truly a functioning arm of the University of Kansas School of Medicine. We in no way envision ourselves as a separate entity in Wichita." The testing evaluations and the board scores from Wichita were compatible with those in Kansas City. What was more, "because we are a youthful program, it still has flexibility."[494]

In 1990, Meek became president of the Kansas Medical Society and, in January 1991, became the fourth dean of KUSM-W. Not only did his outgoing personality, wide achievement in publication and research, and interesting background working with the original Mercury astronauts in the 1960s fit him for the job, but also it cemented the relationship with KU and emphasized that the school at Wichita was here to stay.[495]

Chapter Nine

"Cooperation, Integration, Process"

Meek was in a unique position to bridge the gap with Wichita. Starting as a professor of internal medicine and endocrinology at KUSM, he had moved to the administrative positions of head of the outreach program and then vice chancellor for academic affairs at KUMC. In the latter position, he had reported directly to the executive vice chancellor, Waxman. The dean at KUSM-W in turn reported to Meek, along with four other deans. Meek had therefore been much involved with the Wichita budgets, recruitment of chairs and faculty, and the campus refurbishing. He had, he said, "a good upbringing on the Wichita campus."

He had heard over the years all the rumors and backbiting there was at Kansas City about Wichita. He estimated that, at one time, 90 percent of the faculty at Kansas City would have voted against having anything to do with Wichita "let alone sending our valuable students down there." He was also aware of what he called "rampant paranoia" in the Wichita community about Lawrence and Kansas City and their ambitions, noticing that the television weathermen in Wichita always stood in front of Kansas City when showing the weather map. Many of his colleagues at Kansas City, when he told them he was going to Wichita as a professor of internal medicine, were "very explicit" in saying that this would be Meek's "death knell in academic medicine." The only ones who encouraged him were his enemies.

So what motivated Meek to move? For one thing, the mission of Wichita was central to where medical education was going. There was, Meek said, "political hay to be made from espousing that viewpoint." KU had "lusted after" the federal money that was going to come to campuses focused on primary care and outreach. It was, as Meek put it, "low money bags on the tree." This was also true of funding from the state legislature. KUSM-W had done a good job of establishing the right kind of school, and Meek thought by the late 1980s that it was stable and permanent. The average tenure of a dean in medical schools was about three years, and Wichita deans had lasted longer. The table of organization was clearer than it had been, the curriculum had evolved and was better coordinated with KUMC, the students enjoyed the experience and did well upon graduation, and there was strong support in the Wichita medical community for the enterprise. True, research was still unborn at Wichita, and Meek knew very well that there were members of the legislature who felt there was some sort of "covenant" about Wichita that "thou shalt not do research." There, perhaps, the passage of time would change things.

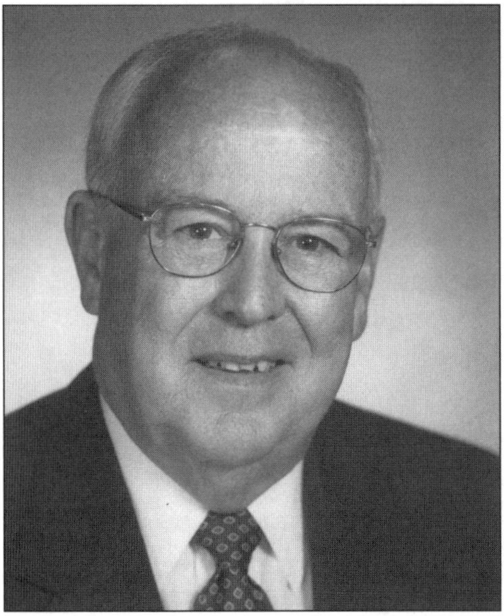

Joseph Meek, M.D.

Meek naturally recognized that there might be resistance in Wichita to an "outsider," and particularly to someone so closely connected with the administration at KUMC, taking over as dean of KUSM-W. It seemed to help immensely, however, that he came first, in 1985, as a department chair and had time to establish himself with the faculty and community before becoming dean.[496] Dr. Frederick Chang, in the Department of Surgery, emphasized that Meek was a "critical dean," in that he was the first "academic-type person" to serve in that position. He understood "what it meant to be an academician" but was also politically savvy. He continued the program of Reals to create a better relationship with Kansas City and with the legislature in Topeka. Part of his strategy was simply presence: talking more with legislators, members of commerce, and officials of Washington departments. By the 1990s, Chang thought, those ties were strong enough that it would "be difficult for Kansas City to do anything negative to this campus," even had it wanted to, and it increasingly did not. Chang, too, was one of those on the faculty who was less enthusiastic about the outreach program and the earlier heavy emphasis at KUSM-W on training for family practice. It was hard for the kind of specialists whom the institution needed to recruit as academic full-time faculty to travel to workshops in Goodland or Harper, Chang thought. As the makeup of the faculty and the nature of the

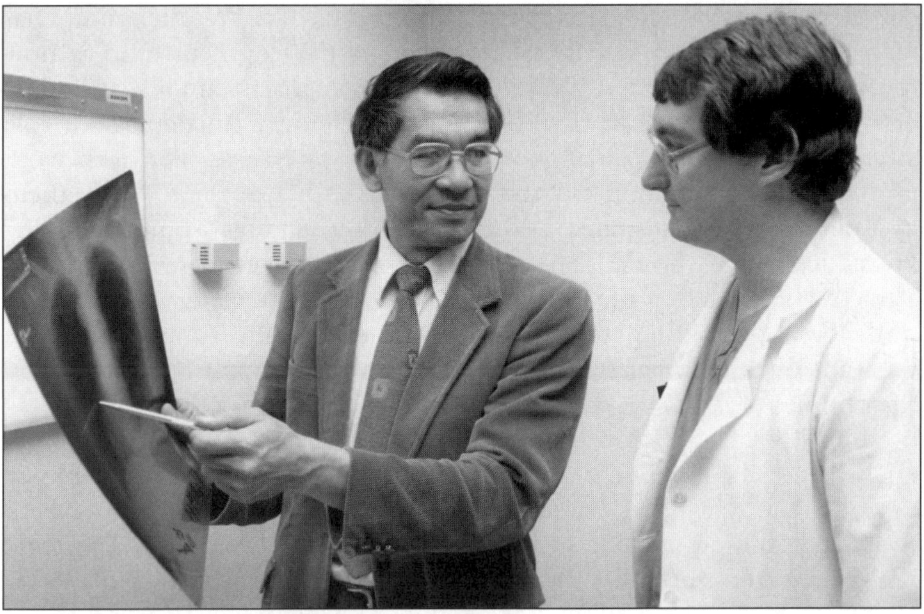

Left: Frederick Chang, M.D.

curriculum changed, that emphasis, while still there, became less overwhelming. KUSM-W became a traditional medical school with a twist, rather than a semi-radical experiment that might eventually have seemed dated and less relevant in the twenty-first century with its changed priorities.[497]

Jerry Slaughter, executive director of the Kansas Medical Society, commented about KUSM-W at the time of Meek's appointment as dean, "I think people in Wichita kind of take it for granted. It's really a kind of model example of how a community of medicine and a community as a whole can embrace and strengthen and bring a special kind of excellence to a medical school endeavor." Dr. Reals said that Meek was "outgoing, affable, friendly, intelligent, and a leader" and thought he would be well accepted. Said a member of the search committee, "He fully knew the scope of this very peculiar thing we call a medical school." Noted another, "He is a very invigorating person to be around. He has a very positive outlook on things; he's thoughtful and kind and you can see why he wanted to be a physician—he's got all the qualities. . . . He likes people he meets and he just is a generally nice man." To boot he was a native Kansan, born in Sabetha. Meek himself commented, "The very thing we think is the hallmark of being a Kansas-trained doctor is distilled right here in Wichita. We absolutely guarantee that if a student comes here on any clinical elective or in any area that there will be a broad, rich clinical experience for that student to see."[498]

Meek himself analyzed the situation. "KUSM-W," he said, "has reached an excellent stabilizing point in its development, and is now recognized as a very credible clinically based medical campus. It is time now to look at new endeavors—a good opportunity to address our role as a major source of primary care physicians for Kansas. We must work in a coordinated fashion to attract students, educate them, place them in good residency programs, and establish them in practice in the state." He added, "We should play a major role in making our community attractive to qualified physicians and then recruit them to our teaching staff. We are not competing, polarizing or separating from Kansas City. We want Wichita to be as strong as it can be. To accomplish that, we need to continue to work together."[499]

In 1994, Meek added a bit to that original statement. He saw the goals then as "cooperation . . . integration . . . process." The school was not, he thought, "an island unto ourselves. We need to develop strategic planning and integrate our mission into the total KU picture. We've matured enough now that we need to be cognizant of where we fit into a statewide effort." Meek praised programs which "provide a continuum of interest in medicine from high school through establishment of a medical practice." All that was needed was more focus on the "nuances of primary care."[500]

Jan Arbuckle headed a community image committee. Its activities included a group of speakers who ran a series of free seminars entitled "Family Challenges in the '90s."[501] In 1992, Van Bush Marketing did an internal image study. It found that the employees thought KUSM-W was doing a good job but three-fourths thought that people in Wichita did not know it. Most also thought the research was not as it should be.[502] In 1994, the school created a speakers' bureau designed to promote KUSM-W's image in the community. Roger Klingman of Wichita High School South trained volunteers using the Toastmasters' "speechcraft" syllabus so that they could address civic groups on the accomplishments of KUSM-W.[503]

Faculty continued to achieve and in the 1990s received more recognition through awards, just as their departments earned similar recognition and endowed professorships were created to allow outstanding faculty to be full-time academics. By 2003, eight Wichita faculty members had won the prestigious University of Kansas Chancellor's award for excellent teaching.[504] Dr. Donna Sweet, of the Department of Internal Medicine, became internationally known for her work in research and treatment relating to HIV/AIDS. In 1993, she received an award from the American Foundation for AIDS research in New York City after having received the Chancellor's Award for

Excellence in Teaching in 1991.[505] In 1994 she received the Crumbine Award from the Kansas Public Health Association for outstanding contribution to public health.[506]

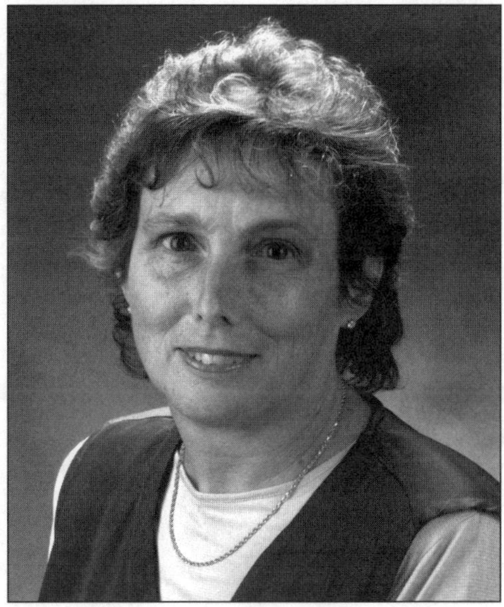
Donna Sweet, M.D.

There continued to be great attention to, and flexibility with, students. This had dated from Hazel Fenske acting rather like a den mother to them in a world that could be stressful and impersonal. Barbara Delhotal recalled that Wichita "stayed more willing to help students to get the kind of experience they are looking for. If you want to tailor an elective it has always been my feeling that the Wichita campus was a lot more student friendly."[507] Chang remembered that the students at KUSM-W seemed happy, while students at Kansas City in general did not seem very happy. Chang's son was at KUSM, and thought that the size and levels of committees there made students perceive that they were a kind of inconvenience.[508] Dr. Hewitt Goodpasture of the KUSM-W faculty in internal medicine had trained at KUSM. His observation was that there were advantages at Kansas City for a certain kind of student and at Wichita for another. Probably on the average, he thought, KUSM provided the better education, but there were two types of students who particularly thrived at Wichita. One was a student who was a bit tentative or non-assertive. That person might very well "fade into the woodwork" at Kansas City. The other type of student who excelled in Wichita was a highly motivated, self-starting, outstanding student who could and would, to some extent, tailor his or her own education and take full advantage of the opportunities in the experience with physicians and hospitals there. Goodpasture's view was that although the two schools became more similar over the years, there was perhaps more load of routine putting in catheters and other university hospital "scut work" for students in Kansas City, while in Wichita there was more time to pursue other things.[509] Finally, one of the weaknesses of KUSM-W, its lack of a strong research focus, may have been helpful to students. While many faculty members, Roberts prominent among them, emphasized that good research was essential to good teaching, the relative lack of pressure to publish at the Wichita campus doubtless left more time to devote to students. Such research as was done, being clinically based, was perhaps more immediately transferable in a practical way to a student.[510]

Meek's only reluctance at becoming dean was that his administrative responsibilities would come at the expense of personal care of patients.[511] Dr. Budig, the KU chancellor, thought, however, that Meek's move into administration was a wise choice. Meek, Budig said, "was the perfect choice to go the school in Wichita." He was, Budig said, an unusual leader who was especially good with students and faculty. Budig commented in 2003, "I always thought he would offer a unique brand of leadership to that operation and history proved that to be the case."[512]

Meek set his agenda for the 1990s quickly. He proposed an expanded curriculum, attention to medical ethics, and more clinical research while continuing to stress primary care. "I think there's an excitement at the medical school here in Wichita," he commented, "and the excitement is because it's a community-based medical school. There isn't the isolation that oftentimes exists in traditional medical schools and the community. Competition for patients, competition in health care delivery—that doesn't exist here because our university hospitals are the community hospitals." Research was basic and not a frill. Said Meek, "The university has some obligation that in the practice of medicine, there's some ability to get trends, ideas, new treatments, evaluation of ongoing therapy—all of that—done. What else is the role of a university if it isn't for that?"[513]

In some ways the world came around to the mission and goals of KUSM-W, just as it became a bit more conventional. RoxAnn Dicker commented in 2003 that "now everyone is trying to do what we were doing twenty years ago."[514] Far from creating some sort of "Marcus Welby" type of kindly general practitioner, the family practice program at KUSM-W familiarized students with a broad range of specialties in order that they might recognize when a specialist was required and what type was needed. In psychiatry, for example, students were not expected to learn to deal with the seriously mentally ill, but to recognize psychiatric symptoms (which were present to some degree in perhaps 40 percent of all cases) and to understand psychological principles. To be aware of that was exactly a follow-up on Dr. Reed's "holistic" approach to analyzing the entire patient. Dr. George Dyke would take students in the evenings to an emergency room to observe and identify the mental issues and how they should be addressed. Otherwise, there might be a tendency to see a person with a cut wrist, and merely fix the wound without asking about the cause.[515] All this, by the 1990s, had become tradition. There was, remembered Dr. Craig Molgaard, who arrived in 1996 to head the new

Masters of Public Health Program, "a fair amount of partnership in different directions," and a sense of history in the day to day activity, a "reflection of continuity with change." The school was small enough that there was good institutional memory, and the community partnership developed slowly but surely. "We are good at it," Molgaard commented, and once the partnership was achieved "it is a pleasure to work within it."[516] And certainly the results began to show. Dr. Sheldon Preskorn observed at the turn of the twenty-first century that although inpatient psychiatric facilities in Sedgwick County had declined from seven to one during the 1990s because of lack of reimbursement by insurance companies for these ailments, KUSM-W had filled the gap well with community interaction with sheriff's and police departments. Although Preskorn recalled the Department of Psychiatry as "cobbled together" based on who was available, he remembered it too as "a very energized" and effective department.

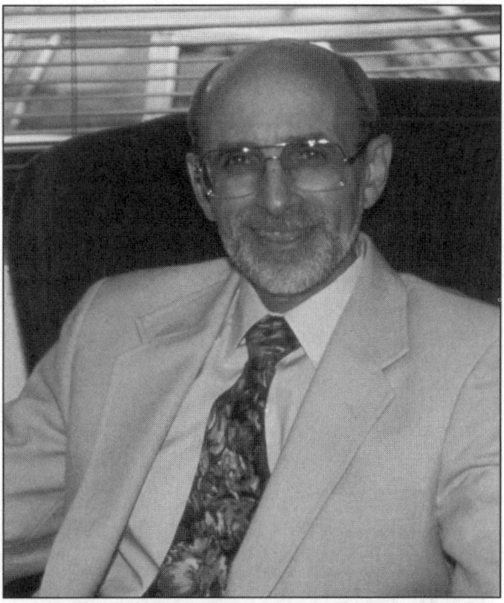

Sheldon Preskorn M.D.

By the turn of the century about 70 percent of the psychiatrists in Sedgwick County were either graduates of the KUSM-W department or members of its faculty.[517] At that same date about half the general and half the orthopedic surgeons in Wichita, as well as three of the four peripheral vascular surgeons and five of the nine plastic surgeons had been trained or had done residencies through KUSM-W. Dr. Alex Ammar, a vascular surgeon who became a member of the KUSM-W faculty in 1982, observed how crucial this was to the quality of medicine in the community. Recruiting specialists

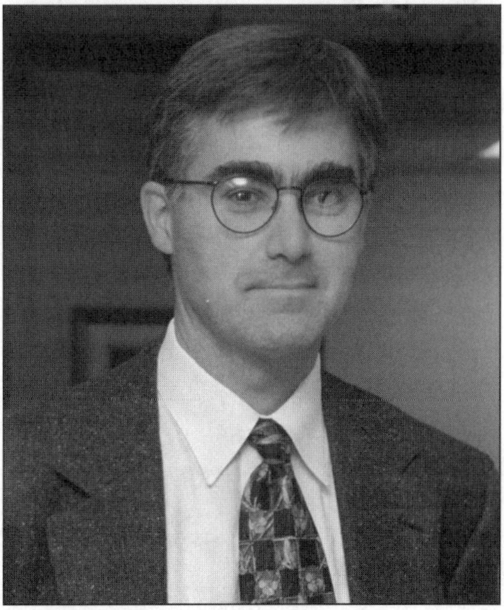

Alex Ammar, M.D.

and sub-specialists was vital. In this, the school helped in two ways. First, outstanding people seemed to be interested in an atmosphere of teaching and research. Second, students who had experience with Wichita and became outstanding practitioners were much more likely to return to Kansas even after a considerable period away for sub-specialty training. The Wichita medical community, Ammar thought, had "matured dramatically," since the 1980s, and the medical school had much to do with that. Without it, he said, "we would risk going back into the '40s and '50s with regard to breadth of specialties and ability to recruit doctors here." Also, in surgery and many other fields, techniques and equipment were constantly changing at an increasing rate. Kidney stones at the turn of the twenty-first century were routinely removed by sound wave lithotripsy, and diagnosed by high-tech imaging, neither of which had been thought of a few years earlier. Therefore, the physician's education had to be more than training in technique. It had to provide the doctor with the ability to reeducate him or herself constantly over a lifetime.[518] And KUSM-W accomplished that. There was no question that it made a big difference.

Internally, the school began to work more smoothly. Jan Arbuckle remembered the "silo mentality" that had existed previously, and the "seamless information technology" that developed in the mid-1990s. Computers were applied more imaginatively, and territorial imperatives within KUSM-W diminished. Laptops and networks were only two of the new and revolutionary electronic innovations.[519] In 1991, KUSM-W bought fifty-eight laptops for students at a cost of $200,000. They could access the KU library and various databases of medical information around the country. This laptop program was thought to be the first in the country. With a seven-pound Memorex 386X notebook with internal modems and fax capability, the student on a rural preceptorship was connected with the entire medical world. Students accessed their assignments and reading lists through their computers by 1992, as well as outlines of medical cases.[520]

There was more formal coordination with Kansas City. Dr. Garold Minns, who had started his connection with KUSM-W as a student in 1975, served as a resident under Dr. Voth, joined the faculty in 1980, and eventually became Associate Dean for Academic and Student Affairs, saw several watershed developments in the 1980s and 1990s in the area of KU relations. First, there was a major revision of the Wichita curriculum in 1985–86. Many people had thought of KUSM-W as, to use Minns's phrase, a "hula-hoop" that would not survive the trend that created it. By 1985, it was clear it would survive. A site visit in the mid-1980s noted that there was one medical school and it gave one degree and there needed to be one curriculum. There could not be an eight-week surgery rotation in Wichita and one of twelve weeks in Kansas City. Therefore, during that period, many meetings with Kansas City faculty resulted in a thorough revision. The by-laws of KUSM were rewritten at the same time by a series of joint committees. In 1992, the two faculties began meeting together regularly, often in Emporia, which was located midway between Wichita and Kansas City. Later the meetings were rotated between Wichita and Kansas City. This contact meant more respect of the faculties for each other, which was particularly advantageous for Wichita. As Minns put it, Kansas City, in that period, learned that Wichita did not have a "pseudo faculty" who just practiced medicine and nothing else. It knew something about education. A second major factor, Minns thought, was the death of Roberts. Roberts had been such a giant and a fixture in the city of Wichita that his passing all by itself changed the flavor of the relationship between the faculty and the school. When Wesley honored Roberts in 1990 with a $250,000 gift to KUSM-W for an endowed professorship in his name, it was not only an appropriate recognition of his massive achievements, but an acknowledgement that he personally would not be around to shake things up anymore. In 1999, George Farha stepped down as the head of surgery. The absence of those two in the daily operations of the school truly marked the end of an era, for better and for worse, but certainly for better in the sense of making KUSM-W less a Wichita institution, and less autonomous *vis a vis* the University of Kansas. The sale of Wesley Hospital accelerated that non-local trend, also. HCA had headquarters in Nashville and was not concerned with historical jealousies between Wichita and Kansas City, or for that matter with the particular ambitions of the city of Wichita.[521] Kansas City felt less threatened and relations were smoother.

Another factor in changes in that direction, not so much emphasized by Minns, but mentioned regularly by others, was the departure of Dr. Douglas Voth. Voth was clearly a true academic, and also a man who believed in the relation of practice to good teaching. He had a strong personality (although certainly no stronger than people like Roberts and Farha) and definite views. His methods inspired some and offended others. When he left, therefore, to be replaced by Dr. Meek as chair of the Department of Internal Medicine, it changed the culture as well as the administration.

Dr. Lauren Welch was an admirer. He described Voth as a "man of unparalleled integrity, a fine teacher and a nurturer of residents and students." But Welch noted, too, that Voth was not a man given to compromise or to bending his program to the interests of the hospital training programs. In some ways his leaving under pressure was a signal to others, some of whom left with him, that Kansas City had prevailed, and that both the idealism that had characterized the early KUSM-W, and the strong influence upon it by practitioners in the community, would be lessened in the future.[522]

Dr. Hewitt Goodpasture, Voth's assistant for some years, was also an admirer and, some thought, the calm "front man" for Voth to put things back together after a disagreement. Goodpasture saw Voth's volatility as a brand of the charisma and determination many early leaders of the school had to have, including Reed, who seemed too mild-mannered on the exterior. Voth, like those others, was determined to involve community physicians in the education program, and called upon them personally when their enthusiasm flagged. Sometimes Voth would involve thirty people in the oral exam at the end of a student rotation, most of them community volunteers. As KUSM-W hired more full-time faculty there was less perceived need for that, and the atmosphere of the place and the tone of the chairs changed.

Goodpasture could see that Voth was "not too diplomatic." He had a strong sense of what the school needed to do, and was a strong leader with a strong sense of mission, but did alienate some through that very determination. Any department chair at KUSM-W had to work with many constituencies, not all of which were individuals, and not all of which were close enough to any personality day by day to have a proper understanding of that person's true motivation and aims. Goodpasture's opinion was that, after ten years of outstanding service, Voth, who was constantly rocking the boat, particularly with some hospitals with which the school was desperate to maintain smooth relations, was a threat to the stability and maturity that a school, grown past the entrepreneurial stage, was now keen to enhance. Idealism drove the place when Voth arrived. It did not so much when he left. Goodpasture's take was that people wear out on idealism: that is simply human nature. They become fatigued with creativity, as much as they do with inferior facilities and low salaries, and ask, "do we have to keep doing this?" Voth, like Reed, did not want to mimic the university structure or create a stifling bureaucracy, but in that he was out of sympathy with the deans at least from Reals on. The new leadership could appreciate innovation, but saw stability as the key to survival in the times and situation in which they found themselves. Voth, therefore, moved on to a very successful career elsewhere where perhaps the parameters were different. His departure, like the other factors about the same time, however, were more evidence of an "end of an era" scenario as the first generation disappeared.

Almost emblematic of the school as "establishment" was the completion of the renovation of its physical plant. And no sooner was that completed than there was a view toward expanding it. In 1990, KUSM-W purchased a two-acre plot of land west of the campus for expansion and developed a twenty-five year site plan. The budget in 1990 was $18 million, but there was hope for much more, especially during what might be Meek's "honeymoon period" as dean. There were thoughts of a student center. The biomedical research facility, with a price tag of $10 million, was still under discussion. Certainly the 100,000 square foot main facility was becoming cramped.[523]

Outreach grew apace also. In 1991, a Primary Care Bridging Plan (later known as the Kansas Bridging Plan) was developed, which helped match new doctors to non-metropolitan areas in Kansas, partly using computers. The start came from a $600,000 grant from the Wesley Foundation—part of the $30 million that foundation gave in the previous five years for medical research and health care in Kansas. Doctors who had completed one year of residency could get up to $5,000 in grant money and $5,000 in community matching funds each year in addition to their residency salary. Each then agreed to maintain a practice in the community equal to the time during which he or she received assistance. Thirty doctors would participate in the next two years in this program.[524] The program attracted the attention of the White House in 1992. Over the objections of the *Wichita Eagle* that the federal government should not be involved in financing such programs, Senator Nancy Kassebaum helped with a bill approved by the U.S. Senate to channel grant money to medical schools that placed students in underserved areas. Lorene Valentine, director of Rural Health Education and Services, the office which administered the Bridging Plan, said, "Other medical schools have come up with their own programs since then, but I think we were the first." KUSM-W students did not go just to medium-sized towns like Salina, Hutchinson, or Garden City. "They're going to places like Quinter, Iola, Fort Scott, Tribune, Seneca. When KUSM-W's Wesley Foundation grant for this Bridging Plan program ran out, the state agreed to step in and financed it for $321,000 a year."[525]

Much was added to the traditional rural health outreach. The traditional job fair continued, now called the Kansas Practice Opportunities Conference. This formalized meeting between medical students and small towns needing doctors was extended to the Kansas City campus as well, and Valentine expanded the Wichita component. In 1994 there were 170 participants. Thirty-seven Kansas towns sent representatives. Seminars and workshops included titles such as "The Real World: What Your Medical Education Didn't Teach You," and "Stress in the Medical Family."[526] In 1993, the Kansas Health Foundation granted $196,718 to fund rotations in rural primary care for internal medicine residents. Called the Primary Care Initiative, the program provided a home, utilities, and living expenses for a resident's family.

The first such resident, Nancy Brecheisen, M.D., who hailed from Eudora, started at the Mitchell County Hospital in Beloit in September 1993. Her supervisor there was Craig Concannon, M.D., who was an associate professor of internal medicine at KUSM-W, a regular preceptor for students there, and himself a 1984 graduate of that institution.[527] There was a videoconference that year which allowed four western Kansas high school student participants in a summer health career program to interview a family physician and a fourth year medical student. One medical student from Hays commented, "When I was in high school, I never even knew a medical student, let alone got a chance to talk to one."[528]

In 1993 also began the Locum Tenens program, which provided backup from the medical school for rural doctors on vacation. Only the largest Kansas counties were barred from applying for this help.[529] Jay Allen, a student who spent four weeks in the fall of 1993 working at the Clay Center Family Physicians office as part of the preceptorship program, said, "I can't see myself living in a big town. It's hard to describe, you just know, you just have a feeling." Dr. Jimmie Browning in Clay Center took Allen to a local high school football game and Allen learned that "the practice of medicine in a small town doesn't stop in the office."[530] The same year, Valentine started a newsletter called *Kansas Connections*, which had an exclusive focus on rural health in Kansas.[531]

Some of this activity went all the way back to the establishment of the College of Health Related Professions at Wichita State University, which had launched the whole KUSM-W project. When Dr. Claud Harwood, the only doctor in Glasco, Kansas, retired in 1992 after thirty-four years, Kansas was ready. Some in town had reservations about the nurse practitioner, Debra Folkerts, an R.N. with advanced training who had begun helping Harwood in 1990. But the town of 500 came to accept her and the system. By 1992 Folkerts saw about 350 patients a month in the region. She was affiliated with Dr. Cary Herl of Concordia, who visited her clinic once a week, and she had the advantage of a two-way video hookup and a network of medium-sized hospitals.

Lorene Valentine commented that this was just the way things were designed to be, but there was a shortage of such mid-level practitioners. There were only 200 licensed in Kansas. And while there were 130 qualified applicants a year to the training program, only thirty could be accepted at KU, WSU, and Fort Hays State University.

Funding came and went, and the proportion of federal, state, and private support varied year by year.[532] It seemed that when the federal government backed off the program, the state stepped in. For example, the Kansas Department of Health and Human Services granted KUSM-W $70,000 in 1993 for community medicine.[533]

Private help slowly came. Much of it was modest. The Southwestern Bell Foundation for Economic Excellence Program kicked in $5,000, for example, for a Practice Opportunity Conference in Wichita in November 1993 sponsored by Rural Health Education and Services at KUSM-W and designed to connect recruiting communities with residents.[534] The activities of The Wesley Foundation, renamed Kansas Health Foundation were, of course, on a different scale. And that scale was to move in the middle of the decade from substantial to definitive in affecting the destiny of KUSM-W.

The Office of Rural Health Education and Services at KUSM-W put on conferences and pizza parties to advance its cause.[535] Private physicians groups developed programs directly. The Galichia Group, in 1994, ran seventy-four clinics a month using two planes and pilots to fly physicians and staff to towns to educate people on heart disease. Dr. Joseph Galichia himself was from a small town in southeast Kansas and had a special appreciation of the problems.[536] An advertisement for Galichia showed a graphic saying "Derby City Limits" with the caption "We Consider This a Vital Sign." The text read: "The way we see it, a person shouldn't have to drive hours and hours to get special medical advice." So Galichia cardiologists were coming to the people.[537] There were varied means to the end. The most important thing was that there was continuity and success in the bridging program and in primary care and public health areas in issues that had led to the creation of KUSM-W in the first place.

Within the community the school escalated its social activity on medical issues. It was a participant, for example, in the move in the early 1990s to replace the coroner's office in Sedgwick County with a more modern system of a medical examiner operating in a forensic center. There was no question that Dr. William Eckert, deputy coroner of Sedgwick County, was one of the outstanding practitioners of his craft in the nation. He had performed 20,000 autopsies in thirty-five years, but the facilities he used, located at the Diplomat Mortuary Service, were, according to Dr. Reals, himself a forensic pathologist of note, "archaic." Reals told the press, "You need photographers; you need toxicologists; you need lab attendants. We don't have any of that stuff. We don't even have a morgue."[538] The effort to create a medical examiner's office succeeded. Late in 1995, Sedgwick County built a $3.4 million forensic science facility right next door to KUSM-W.[539]

The Hunter Health Clinic, an outgrowth of the original KUSM-W connection with the Mid-America All-Indian Center, formed in 1985.

It served over 500 Native American patients a month by 1992 at its clinic on East Central. It was the only federally funded community health center in Kansas, and its president, Bert Steeves, thought it should be a model for other applications, and that health care should be a right. Eighty percent of its patients were below the federal poverty line and more than 90 percent of them would have gone to emergency rooms for care had the clinic not existed. Many were homeless or working poor and the Hunter Clinic received over 20,000 medical visits a year for them. Dr. Walling of KUSM-W arranged a family practice rotation there for medical students that began in the fall of 1992. Then it had a staff of forty-three full-time and ten part-time, and a budget of $2.6 million a year. It was a good example of a community institution, which KUSM-W by no means controlled but clearly had fostered.[540]

Earlier difficulties with hospitals continued to diminish. Hospitals needed the school and vice versa. Sister Sylvia Egan, who retired as chief executive of St. Francis Hospital in 1995, observed, "When you get a university it gets clamped up tight," and she missed the days of more flexibility. However, the bottom line at hospitals was not so healthy in the 1990s as it had been in the 1980s, and the help in funding residencies and handling accreditation was welcome. Strong residencies were good publicity for hospitals. It was a "good omen," Egan remembered, "and showed you had qualified physicians and were sort of a number one hospital."[541] Interestingly, too, hospital requirements led KUSM-W in some directions it wanted to go. For example, the creation of trauma centers at Wichita hospitals required a certain level of clinical research, which had to be provided through KUSM-W.[542]

An important addition to the mission and curriculum of KUSM-W in the early 1990s was the creation of major emphases upon public health and preventive medicine. In 1991, KUSM-W established the Department of Preventive Medicine. This department had an initial goal of establishing a Masters of Public Health (MPH) degree jointly administered with the College of Health Related Professions at Wichita State University. It was, said one internal publication, a strong example, "of how public health, preventive medicine and primary care can be combined to meet the needs of a growing statewide population." A student needed at least one year of work experience as a health professional for admission to the program.[543] A 1993 gift of the Kansas Health Foundation of $1.6 million to endow a public health professorship at Wichita led to a national search for an outstanding person to join the Department of Preventive Medicine.[544] "We see our department as a statewide resource," Dr. S. Edwards Dismuke, department chair, who ultimately filled the endowed professorship in public health position, commented. "We are interested in individual and population approaches to health care delivery; what better population can we have than the entire state?" The other department members were: Drs. Anne Walling, James Early, and Doren Frederickson; Sue Lai, Ph.D.; and Dr. Cramer Reed, who served as a volunteer. Dr. Early noted, "All our faculty members have broad knowledge of preventive medicine. They have expertise in pediatrics, internal medicine, family practice, epidemiology, biostatistics, environmental health, and health care administration. It is the goal of the department to integrate this broad base of knowledge into the systems of primary care and public health that will spell the future of health care in Kansas." Walling thought it was real pioneering. The graduate program was aimed at people already skilled in conventional patient care or administration. "The MPH aims to go beyond teaching classical public health content—it will attempt to create a cadre of individuals in Kansas who share goals and practical skills appropriate to a new way of regarding and working in health." The new department worked with the Kansas Department of Health and Environment on several levels and, as was appropriate, helped organize such statewide initiatives as Operation Immunize to immunize Kansas children under age two.[545]

In 1991, the presidents of KU and WSU agreed to a master's program in public health, which also much complemented the goals in that area of KUSM-W.[546] This program began in earnest in 1996 when Dr. Craig Molgaard arrived as site director. He later became executive director for the program as a whole, which had training sites in Wichita, Lawrence, and Kansas City. He also served eventually as chair of what became known, in 2002, as the Department of Preventive Medicine and Public Health at KUSM-W and also as Associate Dean for Research at that institution.[547] Dr. S. Edwards Dismuke, who came in 1991 as the national expert in public health and preventive medicine that the Kansas Health Foundation grant had recruited, not only established the department, but later became dean of KUSM-W as a whole. Dr. Dismuke had initially taken a job at KUSM in Kansas City, but Wichitans convinced him that there was an opportunity in Wichita to create a program that was "particularly noted and not second fiddle." At the time, there was $1.5 million for the professorship, about the same amount for a building, another $1 million for faculty development in the area, and $3 million for the Masters in Public Health program. These maneuvers jump-started the state of Kansas into going from a place with few who were trained in public health to one of the outstanding states in the nation in this field in a matter of about five years.[548] There could be no better illustration of how good KUSM-W had become at coordination, adaptation, and cooperation, and of the benefits of those skills.

Some sense of the level and range of activities of departments may be gained by summarizing the annual reports for the early 1990s of just one of them, albeit perhaps the most central one for judging the success of KUSM-W's special mission, the Department of Family and Community Medicine. The summary may have some of the characteristics of a "laundry list," but to those living the history at the institution there was drama and meaning in all the details. And the smallest project became substantial as KUSM-W grew up. It was no longer the shadow of one man, but the lives and efforts of many intelligent and energetic people.

There were seven faculty members in that department in 1990: Dr. Andrew Barclay was the chair and Dr. Anne Walling the vice chair. Other members were Dr. Robert Haskins, Dr. E.P. Donatelle, Dr. Sudha Elangovan, Ken Kallail, Ph.D., and Randy Rehbiel, LSCSW. This group was the so-called central faculty located at the former E.B. Allen facilities. In addition there was staff at Wesley Family Practice, St. Joseph Family Practice, St. Francis Family Practice, and Smoky Hill Family Practice in Salina. That year the department sponsored the ninth annual Family Practice Continuing Education Conference at the Marriott Hotel. There were thirty-seven research projects, on such topics as why physicians change practice location, the educational benefits of moonlighting, drug prophylaxis for migraine headaches, and antibiotic use for the elderly. Department goals included: to foster family medicine among students, to define rewards for volunteer faculty, to maintain the individuality of residencies while eliminating intradepartmental competition, to develop a rotation faculty preceptorship and share faculty expertise as co-teachers, to understand the difficulties related to developing and maintaining a commitment to the department by residents and faculty, to establish a department governance committee, and to develop a competency-based curriculum. In the academic year 1990–91 the department established the E.P. Donatelle Student Scholarship Fund. There was a collaborative program

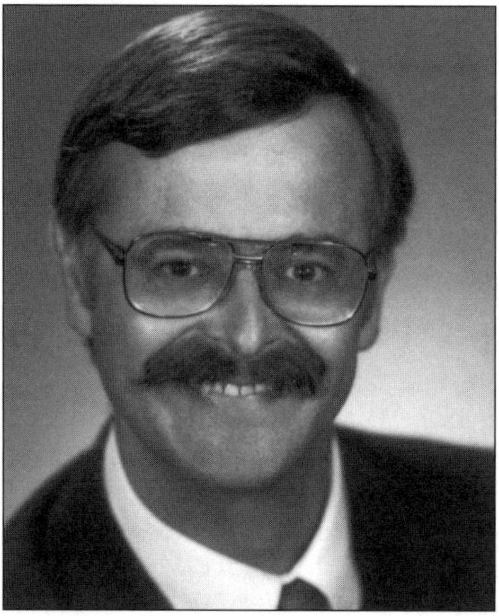

Andrew Barclay, M.D.

with Kansas State University to develop an undergraduate curriculum in rural health linked to the Bridging Plan. The curriculum would emphasize agricultural medicine and rural health care research and would have as a goal to develop skills in assisting rural communities to create and maintain appropriate health care delivery systems. The predoctoral program of the department in that period provided four programs and contributed an Introphase course called "Introduction to Clinical Medicine" for entering juniors. The department and KUSM-W in 1990–91 were awarded a grant of $127,000 from the Department of Health and Human Services to improve the rural preceptorship program. Research projects included "Physician Staffing Responsibilities in Small Rural Hospitals." Students participated in care of over 250 patients on average during their family practice clerkship, and experienced teaching that was reorganized regularly to better emphasize clinical problem-solving and the "development of skills appropriate to 'real world' patient care." The department modified timing of classroom activities to maximize time in patient care and with community preceptors. Grading procedures changed to place greater emphasis on clinical performance and a formal case presentation, though "in an attitudinal based specialty. Evaluation may have to remain highly subjective."

In the preceptorships, the department tried to place students in "centers of excellence" of modern rural practice with new sites in 1990–91 of Council Grove, Clay Center, and Syracuse. These were modeled on the early experiments at Harper, although Harper had to be shut down because of the closing of the practice there through which KUSM-W had worked. Literature searches of rural preceptorship programs in other states showed that they tended "to be long-established courses which emphasize experience but have little structure and uncertain valuative mechanisms." The department in Wichita, however, had learned from the history of its parent institution the importance of combining experience with a strong academic structure.

Twelve of forty-two KUSM-W graduates "matched" in 1990–91 to enter family practice residencies. Overall, about a third of the class had chosen family medicine careers at a time when the national average was only 10 percent. By 1995, that proportion had reached 42 percent of the graduating class. "This allows Wichita to claim to be the most successful program in the country and a major contributor to the growing reputation of the University of Kansas as a leader in Primary Care Education. . . . The 'Wichita model' of clinical experience with a community preceptor, complemented by an integrated program of classroom activities, has been recognized and copied by other medical schools." In the 1991–92 academic year, the Smoky Hill Residency Program received a $127,000 grant from the Department of Health and Human Services to improve the communication and counseling skills of residents. In 1993–94, fifteen of forty-five KUSM-W graduates entered family practice residencies, and eleven of the 1994 residency graduates chose to practice in rural Kansas, the highest number in many years.

Medical students as well as residents seemed much interested in family practice. Senior students spent four weeks in a community preceptorship in one of the three primary care specialties (internal medicine, family practice, pediatrics). In 1990–91, thirty-one students, or 67 percent of the class, chose a family practice placement. A required clerkship in geriatrics, administered jointly by the Departments of Family and Community Medicine and of Internal Medicine, was added to student rotations in 1991. Students and faculty both valued the clerkship enough that there was considerable agitation to extend it, which happened in 1995 when the family practice rotation went to eight weeks. Students had an active Family Practice Interest Group.

The ongoing hypertension-testing program continued to have huge impact, while a focus on African-Americans had led, by 1991, to 5,000 people in this group in Sedgwick County alone being screened for high blood pressure and cholesterol levels by 145 volunteers working through local churches and supervised by department members.

The department worried that its salaries had dropped to low levels when compared with peers nationally. But a high proportion of the class continued to choose family practice residencies and a high proportion of these ended up practicing in rural Kansas. In 1993–94, new doctors from KUSM-W went into family practice at Colby, Wamego, Sterling, Salina, Pratt, Marion, Fort Scott, Atchison, and Great Bend. Grant success was strong. The KUSM-W Medical Practice Association received $1 million from the Public Health Service to develop a federally qualified health center in Wichita to provide care for the underserved. This became the Wichita Primary Care Center (WPCC). It started providing services in the spring of 1994 with a staff of an internist, a physician's assistant, five internal medicine residents, and a family physician. It provided indigent patients with care on a sliding fee scale. "The value of Family Practice has been recognized increasingly around the nation," noted the 1993–94 departmental report. "Family Medicine is becoming part of the mainstream. Our faculty are involved at the highest level and recognized for their innovative . . . leadership."[549]

But it was more than a single department that received recognition beyond Wichita. It was the whole enterprise that had started so tentatively in the late 1960s and was by the 1990s such a key element of the University of Kansas as well as the health care system of Kansas itself. According to *U.S. News & World Report*, in 1992 the University of Kansas was ranked among the top ten medical schools in the nation focusing on primary care.[550] In public health programs, it has ranked as high as second.[551] Of about 900 active physicians in Sedgwick County, KUSM-W paid about 100 of them to be on the faculty and there were 550 or so volunteers. Thus, about two-thirds of the doctors in the county participated in the medical school somehow. About 90 percent of them belonged to the Medical Society of Sedgwick County, contrasted with about 30 percent in Kansas City. There were 300 more volunteers for KUSM-W around the state outside Wichita, making over 800 highly qualified volunteers in all. This was unusual and very effective at accomplishing certain things.[552]

Chapter Ten

KANSAS CONNECTIONS

The year 1995 was one of deserved celebration for KUSM-W. It announced the construction of a 30,000 square foot, $3.5 million addition to its facilities. This was to have two wings, one for the Kansas Health Foundation Center for Primary Care and the other for the Daniel K. Roberts Center for Research. The latter facility included new headquarters for the Women's Research Institute, which had gained an international reputation in growth-factor regulation of ovarian function, biochemistry and physiology of pregnancy-associated proteins, the effects of AIDS in pregnant mothers, mechanism of action of protein hormones, molecular aspects of implantation and proteins, molecular aspects of implantation and early fetal development, and steroid biochemical characterization of tumor development. Its scientists had published 100 papers in a decade, and Dr. Brooks Keel of the institute was the Daniel Roberts Distinguished Professor of Obstetrics and Gynecology at KUSM-W. Grants for the new buildings came from the Kansas Health Foundation, the federal government, and the Roberts family.[553]

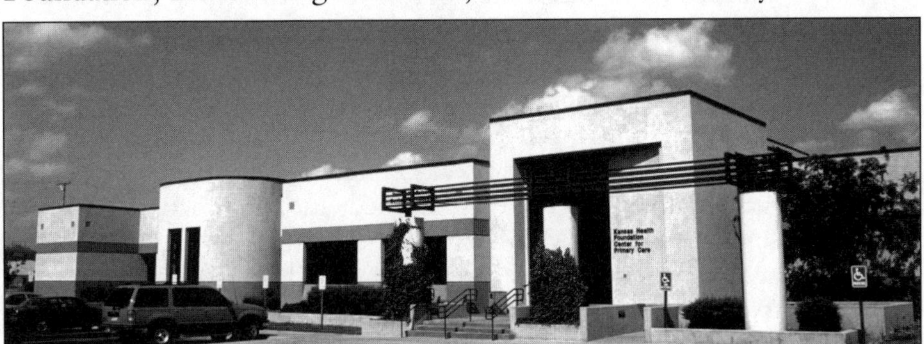

The Daniel K. Roberts Center for Research and
the Kansas Health Foundation Center for Primary Care.

At the same time, there was recognition of the twentieth anniversary of the School. The theme was "Building on the Past—Focused on the Future."[554] The *Wichita Eagle* editorial on the commemoration was entitled "Healthy Story."[555]

That same year, 1995, Dr. Cramer Reed, "the gentleman activist," celebrated his seventy-ninth birthday, still jogging six days a week and climbing 14,000-foot peaks. "Whoever coined the term 'active aging,'" the newspaper wrote, "must have had Cramer Reed in mind." His latest project was Larksfield Place, a different sort of retirement community. For his work there he won the 1994 Trustee of the Year award from the American Association of Homes for the Aging. He also helped develop Shepherd's Centers, a non-profit interfaith organization providing programs for the aging. Reed described himself as "peripatetic." He quipped, "I don't know that they'll really remember me for anything, except that he had occupational instability." Dr. Joseph Meek called him "a treasure."

It was a time for nostalgia about Reed's role in KUSM-W. "I'm sure he didn't do it alone," Meek commented, "but the man who essentially had to lead it was Cramer Reed." Although Reed was quiet, Meek, when he first met him, knew not only that he was "formidable," but found "this man immediately made his presence known as a quality person." He was ahead of his time, Meek thought, and his models were "germane, relevant, appropriate for today's practice of medicine." Jack Davis of Wesley added, "I can't conceive of anyone . . . who would not have some admiration for him."[556]

In 1997, Reed at age eighty-one, became vice chair of the Good Death project to bring local health care workers and community leaders together on an often-neglected topic. Dying, he said in a newspaper interview, was just a matter of cells wearing out, "another event in the scheme of things." Reed was a member of the Hemlock Society, which promoted the right of terminally ill patients to plan their deaths and of physicians to help them. "It's probably easier for me," Reed commented. "I believe in God, I think I believe in a heaven. I'm not sure I'd go so far as to say I know where it is, but I do believe in a hereafter. Death is not an end; it's another stage."[557] That was vintage Cramer Reed—the same concern for the humanistic aspects of medicine that had led to the Introphase seminars at KUSM-W back in the 1970s.

It was important indeed that the model for KUSM-W had been and continued to be sound. The 1990s was clearly another age of rapid change in medicine. Dwight Allen of the Medical Society of Sedgwick County noted that partly do to forced Medicaid write-offs on fees, individual practitioners were disappearing in favor of groups of physicians. More than 30 percent of doctors nationwide were already in groups, and Allen thought that managed care would escalate this trend.[558] Some physician groups were even competing with hospitals through specialized surgery clinics and outpatient facilities. Many doctors, said Dr. Joseph Galichia, "don't want to deal with hospitals and the bureaucracies managing them." Market forces, he thought, would determine the future shape of things.[559] Physicians, the local paper said, were "contracting, merging, aligning—and crossing their fingers that their decisions will prove profitable over time." Hospitals also changed, including a merger of the Wichita Catholic hospitals.

Medical schools were faced with the question of how best to prepare their students for "the increasingly uncertain health care environment of tomorrow." KUSM-W was in a good position to adjust. Jan Arbuckle, associate dean for administration, in a 1996 interview, explained that a strength was that there was no university-owned medical center in Wichita. KUSM-W invited "selected community stakeholders" in July 1996 to a daylong planning retreat to discuss the details of the adjustment. Among items discussed was that KUSM-W was too small to contract with large insurance companies, that the patient pool for the practice association that was supplementing salaries there might dry up, that the merged Catholic hospitals could lure away faculty members as medical directors of their programs, and that the contracting of the school might change. KUSM-W by that time was operating psychiatric and multi-specialty primary care clinics on its campus, an internal medicine clinic at Via Christi Regional Medical Center—St. Joseph campus, and a pediatric clinic at Wesley Medical Center. Managed care could cause all this. However, the school was ready. As Arbuckle put it, "We can't wait until something changes at the federal level . . . not while the changes are occurring every day here."[560]

The legacy, however, was much enhanced by new funding, and particularly by the funding from the Kansas Health Foundation. In 1994, the Kansas Health Foundation asked KUSM to submit a proposal to develop the Primary Care Physician Education (PCPE) Project. Over 100 faculty members, legislators, and administrators worked on the plan over a six-month period, the goal being to create "an environment in Kansas that supports the training of primary care physicians and increases the likelihood that primary care residency graduates will remain in practice in the state." It targeted the most promising rural high school and college students "for exposure to opportunities in primary care medicine." The curriculum changed, the primary care facilities were expanded, physicians collaborated with basic scientists and medical specialists, and nursing and allied health professionals were consulted to promote "a team approach to medical care."[561] The resulting grant of $15 million, made in the spring of 1995, was the largest ever given to the KU Endowment Association.[562]

The PCPE project immediately developed a slide show called "A Career in Medicine" for showing to high schools across the state, organized a collaborative practice task force to better coordinate with other health care professionals, and worked on the curriculum. An internal committee, called the "Big Ten" because it had ten members, performed strategic planning to establish at the school what was called the "gold standard for community-based medical education in primary care." It met as often as three times a month, and it found that its planning helped unify the campus. Wrote Dean Meek: "People are beginning to look at the medical school as a campus and not as individuals with different agendas."[563] Dr. Anne Walling added: "We want to make our state a primary care power in the United States. When people think of quality primary care education, we want them to think of Kansas."[564]

The dean of KUSM said this grant represented "a very major shift in the culture of this institution to make primary care education the centerpiece." Said another doctor in Kansas City: "We'll get to see clinical medicine sooner, and in a primary care setting in the real world" instead of the "glitz and glamour of a (major) hospital. If a medical student spends his entire education in a hospital, frankly the prospect of going back alone to a community of 10,000 can be frightening."[565] Dr. Daniel Hollander of KUMC predicted that in the next five years there would come to exist in Kansas "the medical equivalent of [agricultural] cooperative extension offices. . . . Medical students will leave their classrooms to study one-on-one with physicians in small towns and inner city neighborhoods." The ratio between specialists and primary care doctors would change. There would be a school without walls, and "the plan will revolutionize what we teach, how we teach, and where we teach."[566] These were insights that KUSM-W had promoted for twenty years.

The Kansas Health Foundation helped in many other ways. In the mid-1990s, it turned its attention from developing a major basic science biomedical research center in Wichita to promoting public health. KUSM-W had been a partner with Wichita State University in the earlier initiative, but doubtless, given its mission and history, benefited even more from the change in focus.[567] The new buildings, largely funded by the Health Foundation, have been mentioned. These changed the look of the campus as they were completed in 1996. But there were many smaller, but important gifts. The year of the major grant in 1995, for example, the Health Foundation gave $42,000 to allow the Hays Medical Center to be the first in the nation to offer routine home health care via interactive television. Thirty interactive telemedicine systems were installed and operated at no charge to patients.[568] The author's brother-in-law, who lived in the tiny western Kansas town of Plainville, was diagnosed at Hays for a rather unusual non-Hodgkin's Lymphoma using this system to consult with major oncology centers around the country. Treatment was successful.

Endowed and distinguished professorships multiplied, reflecting increased prestige. Dr. Dismuke continued as Kansas Health Foundation Distinguished Professor in Public Health.[569] In 2000, Dr. Douglas Woolley of the Department of Family and Community Medicine became the Delos V. Smith Professor in Community Geriatrics, another endowed chair.[570] In 2001, Dr. Douglas Horbelt became the Daniel K. Roberts Professor of Obstetrics and Gynecology.[571] In 2002, Dr. Sechin Cho became the Wesley Medical Center Endowed Professor of Pediatrics.[572] Since these professorships often required $500,000 to fund, and since the recipients were the result of a national search, both the existence of the professorships and the fact that they were filled by people already teaching at KUSM-W was a tribute to the quality of the institution. And that was reflected also by honors paid to departments and programs. The Masters of Public Health program, for example, in the early twenty-first century, regularly was ranked in the top ten among all programs and in the top two among public university programs in its special area.[573]

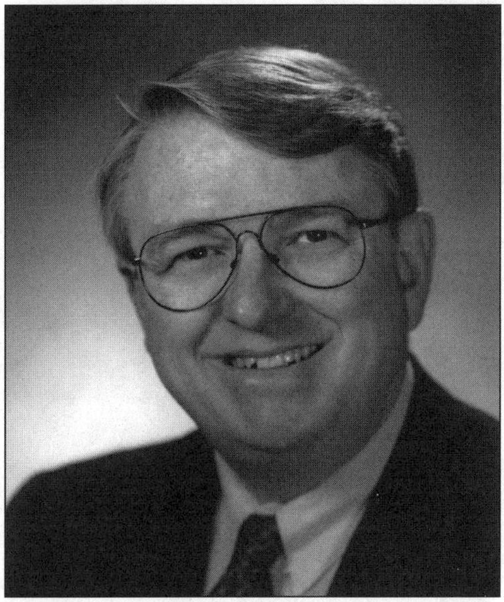

Douglas Horbelt, M.D.

Certainly there was adjustment to change as there always had been. Assessing the situation in the spring of 1996, KUSM-W could boast that 900 had graduated from that institution. Over 60 percent had chosen primary care specialties and half were currently practicing in Kansas.[574] Eighty-seven percent of the students in the Kansas Bridging Plan were staying in the state.[575] True, the move toward managed care was a challenge, as was the general "turbulence in the health care industry." And it was the job of medical schools to prepare them for that uncertain

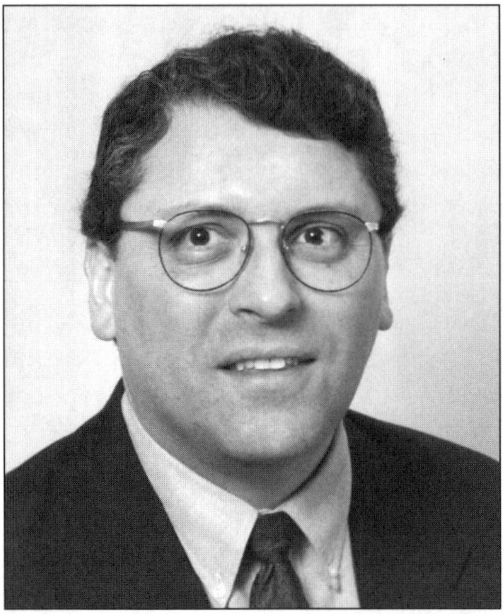

Rick Kellerman, M.D.

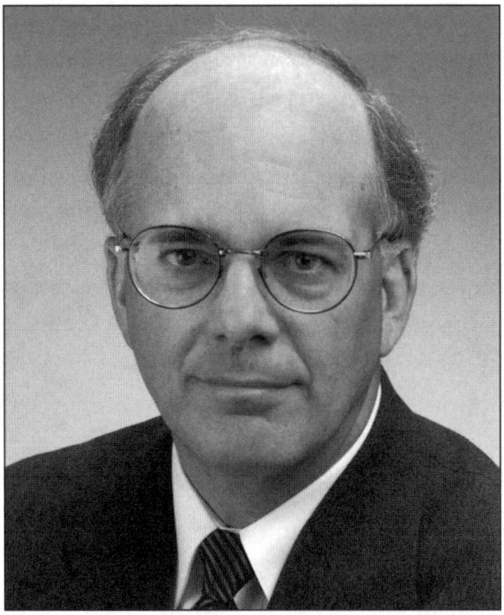

Dr. S. Edwards Dismuke, Dean, KUSM-W

future. Dr. Rick Kellerman, who became chair of the Department of Family and Community Medicine in 1996, said, "The former chairman of a large automotive manufacturer once said that 'the winds of change are blowing so fast that one needs nerves of steel . . . just to be neurotic!'" Something that, Kellerman added, was very true for his department.[576]

One major part of the strategic planning at KUSM-W was a Community Health Assessment Project done by Dr. S. Edwards Dismuke, chair of the Department of Preventive Medicine and Public Health at KUSM-W. The study involved 1,000 phone interviews and compiled a list of over 300 agencies and organizations that provided health care in Wichita. It showed, among other things, that health care costs were rising two or three times faster than other things. This was not a new problem but continued to be a serious one. The medical school used the study to rethink how it cared for the uninsured and the indigent and kept a close eye on the physician mix. The study showed there was not a gross excess of physicians in Kansas, as there were coming to be in some places, and there was about the right mix of primary care physicians, thanks partly to the activities of twenty years of KUSM-W. However, they still were not all in the places that society needed them most to be.[577]

In 2000, Dean Meek, at age seventy, announced he would resign in 2001. He quipped that deans should think about retiring after eight years on the job and act after ten so they could avoid being thrown out after twelve. He said he was proudest at following in his predecessors' footsteps in fitting KUSM-W into the community. "I worked very hard to make sure medical education wasn't done as kind of a contract with the community, but that we *are* the community."[578]

When Meek actually departed from office in the spring of 2001, to be replaced as dean by Dr. Dismuke, he made a few of his patented comments about the state of affairs at his institution. The "Road to Academic Success," in Wichita, he said, had had three phases. The first was the Cramer Reed years, which "involved literally building a campus in an academic wilderness." At that time, there was uncertainty about what role the new school would play. "One thing that was definite, however, was that Wichita demanded a firm academic foundation for whatever was conceived. The problem was, no one knew how to do that." Reed was the pioneer. "The path had been laid out. It wasn't a four-lane highway exactly, but the road the medical school would travel was at least clearly delineated." The second stage was Dr. William Reals. In that era, Meek said, "we had some stability; we had built that four-lane highway." The school was up and running and internal refinements had to be made. "By the 1980s," Meek opined, "there was no doubt that this was a complete medical campus, not just a site for piecemeal rotations from Kansas City. What we had here was a genuine clinical campus." The 1990s began the third stage. There were additional refinements required by the accreditation boards, and of course the building program. "We were approaching expressway status."[579]

Observers agreed that in losing Meek "rural Kansas will be saying good-bye to a great friend and advocate." The small towns, Meek said, were a natural Wichita constituency, and KUSM-W, "strongly entrenched," was evaluated on its own merit and not just as a satellite of Kansas City.[580]

Dr. Dismuke agreed on the direction, no matter what the ups and downs of financing. "Doctors have great ideas to improve the health of the community," he said. "I am interested in helping communities focus on relationships that produce win-win situations." Dismuke was a runner and tennis player with lots of energy, and, maybe more important, was perhaps the only medical school dean in the nation with a specialty in, and experience with, preventive medicine and public health.[581] Early in 2003, he said that even in a year when the budget had to be cut by 7 percent, there was a strong sense of mission. The budget crisis "strengthens and focuses us," he said. "It forces us to determine what our real priorities are." Priorities included strengthening research and responding to accreditation initiatives at the graduate level.[582] That year, KUSM-W welcomed fifty-four new medical students, eight new Masters of Public Health students, and seventy new resident physicians.[583]

Total graduates were, by then, about 1,300, and the campus included over 128,000 square feet. It had 124 full- and part-time paid faculty and 117 staff. There were 750 volunteer faculty and, as always, they were essential to the success and spirit of the place. Its community presence was much more elevated than ever before, involving co-sponsorship of numerous media-based educational series on medicine. Nearly 800 health care professionals benefited that year from seven major conferences coordinated through KUSM-W's Division of Postgraduate Education. No one visiting the facilities would have any inkling that urine smells, bird problems, or leftover pizzas had ever plagued the organization. In fact, in 2003, KUSM-W had an annual budget of over $21 million and was well placed to celebrate its thirtieth anniversary in the year 2005.

More than eighty people agreed to be interviewed for its history. While their perspectives were various, to a person they were impressed by the point, its prospects, and what it had overcome to reach the place where it has now arrived.[584] "You may have had a rocky takeoff," the *Wichita Eagle* commented, "but you're flying high now."[585]

AFTERWORD

This exceptional historical study by Craig Miner, Ph.D., graphically illustrated how the first three decades of our medical school have helped to shape our future vision.

In this volume, Miner captured how we primarily emphasize the teaching of physicians. Our focus has been one of educating future physicians in the primary care disciplines, in surgery, and in obstetrics and gynecology, while exposing them to the sub-specialty clinical practice environment found in among our local facilities and providers.

As you have read, we are a community-based medical school, not residing in a university hospital or employing a large, full-time academic faculty, but instead, partnering with local medical centers to create our teaching base. In fact, 75 percent of the practicing physicians in this community help us teach our medical students and residents, educating these future physicians in a highly successful, real-world setting.

Beyond being community based, we have established ourselves as a community-oriented organization. Through our numerous partnerships, we assist our city, county, local hospitals, and medical society in assessing area health and health care needs; we assure the high quality delivery of medical care and public health to all of our citizens; and we work to address the health policy needs of our community.

These basic methods of assessment, assurance, public health, and health policy development have come to define what community orientation means and will continue to drive our efforts to carry out our mission of educating doctors and public health professionals for Kansas.

Activities like these have shown us the importance of high quality research in the education of doctors and public health specialists. Therefore, in the days before us, we will be placing more emphasis on applied research in clinical medicine, in health services, and in community or public health. We see this new area of concentration as highly relevant to the continued improvement of local medical care for individual patients and our community as a whole.

With the past covered so eloquently by Dr. Miner in this book, we look forward to the future and our ever-increasing role as the premier center for community-oriented medical education, scholarship, patient care, service, and research in Kansas and beyond.

—Dr. S. Edwards Dismuke
Dean, University of Kansas School of Medicine-Wichita

Notes

—Chapter One—

1. For general trends see Frank Campion, *The AMA and US Health Policy Since 1940* (Chicago: Chicago Review Press, 1984). For the background in medical education see Kenneth Ludmerer, *Time to Heal: American Medical Education from the Turn of the Century to the Era of Managed Care* (New York: Oxford University Press, 1999). William Mallon, Mandy Lieu, Robert Jones, Michael Whitcomb, *Mini-Med: The Role of Regional Campuses in U.S. Medical Education* (Washington, DC: Association of American Medical Colleges, 2003. Background for medicine in Kansas may be found in Thomas Bonner, *The Kansas Doctor: A Century of Pioneering* (Lawrence: University Press of Kansas, 1959).
2. Ludmerer, *Time to Heal*, 180–81, 183, 198, 211, 215–16.
3. Interview, Craig Miner with Dr. Gayle Stephens, Feb. 2, 2003.
4. Ibid.
5. Crumbine's autobiography, *Frontier Doctor* (Philadelphia: Dorrance & Co., 1948) is both highly readable and informative.
6. Dr. Rick Kellerman, ed. *In Their Own Words: Stories About the Origin of Family Medicine Education at the University of Kansas School of Medicine in Wichita and Affiliated Residencies* (n.p.: Kansas Academy of Family Physicians Foundation, 1999), ix, 5.
7. Sources for the history of the University of Kansas School of Medicine are Lawrence Larsen and Nancy Hulston, *The University of Kansas Medical Center: A Pictorial History* (Lawrence: University Press of Kansas for the University of Kansas Medical Center, 1992); Ralph Major, M.D., *An Account of the University of Kansas School of Medicine* (Lawrence: University of Kansas Medical Alumni Association, n.d. [1955]; Helen Sims, *The Wahl Years at the University of Kansas Medical Center, 1919–1948* (Lawrence: University of Kansas Alumni Association, 1983); Stanley Friesen and Robert Hudson, *Kansas School of Medicine: Eyewitness Reflections on its Formative Years* (Kansas City: SR Friesen, 1996); Clyde Griffin, *The University of Kansas: A History* (Lawrence: University Press of Kansas), 1974.
8. *Sunflower*, Nov. 20, 1972; *Wichita Eagle*, Feb. 3, 1972; *Medical Society of Sedgwick County News*, Feb. 3, 1972, clippings file, University of Kansas School of Medicine-Wichita archives. (Hereafter cited as KUSM-W archives).
9. Craig Miner, *Studying to Care: A History of the Wesley Medical Research Institutes, 1949–1999* (Wichita: WMRI, 2000), 14–15.
10. Larsen and Hulston, *The University of Kansas Medical Center: A Pictorial History*, 131, 140.

11. Griffin, *The University of Kansas*, 607–610.
12. Dr. Ernest Crow, "Garfield University and the First Medical School in Wichita," *Kansas Medicine* vol., 96, no. 3 (Fall 1995): 114–16.
13. Craig Miner, *A History of the Medical Society of Sedgwick County: The Modern Era* (Wichita: Medical Society of Sedgwick County, 2003), 38.
14. Miner, *Studying to Care*, 14–15. Miner, *Medical Society*, 41. Interview, Craig Miner with Dr. Ernest Crow, Jan. 14, 2003.
15. *Bulletin of the Sedgwick County Medical Society* (May 1952), 11.
16. Ibid., (July 1952), 11.
17. Interview, Craig Miner with Dr. Stan Friesen, May 19, 2003. Major, *Kansas School of Medicine*, 145.
18. Interview, Craig Miner with Dr. Lew Purinton, Mar. 24, 2003.
19. Friesen and Hudson, *Kansas School of Medicine*, 170.
20. Booz, Allen & Hamilton to Rep. Rex Borgen, May 15, 1968 in Booz, Allen & Hamilton, Inc., "A Plan for the Development of Health Resources. State of Kansas," 3 vols. (n.p.: Kansas Dept. of Economic Development, 1968), I, xii.
21. The recommendations are in ibid. vol. 1, 64.
22. Dr. Emory Lindquist to Dr. Clarke Wescoe, June 13, 1968, Chancellor's Papers, Series 2/12/5, Dept. Correspondence 1968/69, box 3, University Archives, Spencer Library, University of Kansas.
23. "Paramedical Education Development (a working document)," typescript, May 14, 1968, box 45, file folder 1, Clark Ahlberg Papers, WSU archives, Special Collections, Wichita State University.
24. Dr. Emory Lindquist to Dr. Clarke Wescoe, June 13, 1968, ibid.
25. Dr. George Wolf to Dr. Clarke Wescoe, Aug. 7, 1968, ibid., file folder 3.
26. Dr. Clarke Wescoe to Dr. George Wolf enclosing report, Nov. 8. 1967, Chancellor's Papers, Series 1/12/5, Department Correspondence 1967–68, box 9, University Archives, Spencer Library, University of Kansas.
27. Dr. Clarke Wescoe to Dr. George Wolf, July 1, 1968, ibid., box 3.
28. Dr. Emory Lindquist to Dr. Clarke Wescoe, June 17, 1968, ibid.

—Chapter Two—

29. Friesen and Hudson, *The Kansas School of Medicine*, 8.
30. Dr. George Wolf to Dr. Clarke Wescoe, Aug. 7, 1968, box 45, file folder 3, Clark Ahlberg Papers, WSU archives, Special Collections, Wichita State University.
31. Dr. George Wolf to Dr. Clarke Wescoe, Oct. 30, 1968, Chancellor's Papers, Series 2/12/4, Department Correspondence 1968/69, University Archives, Spencer Library, University of Kansas.
32. For the general history of Wichita State see Craig Miner, *Uncloistered Halls: The Centennial History of Wichita State University* (Wichita: WSU Endowment Association, 1995).
33. Miner, *Uncloistered*, 286–87.
34. Friesen and Hudson, *Kansas School of Medicine*, 171, 175.
35. Miner, *Uncloistered*, 321.
36. Interview, Craig Miner with Dr. John Breazeale, Feb. 5, 2003.
37. *Wichita Eagle & Beacon*, Apr. 26, 1969, clippings file, KUSM-W archives.
38. Miner, *Uncloistered*, 291, 318.
39. Interview, Craig Miner with Dr. George Platt, Mar. 12, 2003; Miner, *Uncloistered*, 302–07.

40. Dr. Jack Walker, "A Proposed College of Health Related Professions, Wichita State University, Feasibility Study, August 1969," Walker to Ahlberg introductory letter, box 45, file folder 3, Clark Ahlberg Papers, WSU archives, Special Collections, Wichita State University.
41. Ibid., 2.
42. Ibid., 1–2, 7–8, 22.
43. Ibid., 30.
44. Ibid., 37.
45. Booz, Allen & Hamilton, "A Plan," I, 51.
46. Walker, "A Proposed College," 37.
47. Ibid., 40.
48. Ibid., 39.
49. See especially the section by Dr. Stephens in Kellerman, ed. *In Their Own Words*, 227–28.
50. Interview, Craig Miner with Dr. Gayle Stephens, Feb. 3, 2003.
51. Dr. Ernest Crow, "The Early History of the University of Kansas School of Medicine-Wichita. Department of Internal Medicine," typescript in KU School of Medicine-Wichita archives.
52. Interview, Craig Miner with Dr. Ernest Crow, Jan. 14, 2003.
53. Dr. Clark Ahlberg to Dr. Cramer Reed, Feb. 19, 1970, file 1B1, KUSM-W archives.
54. "Reflections, Charles E. Brackett, Jr., M.D." in Friesen and Hudson, *Kansas School of Medicine*, 27.
55. Dr. Clark Ahlberg to Dr. George Wolf, Dec. 5, 1969, Cramer Reed personal papers.
56. *MSSC News* (Mar. 1970), clippings file, KUSM-W archives. Interview, Craig Miner with Hazel Fenske, Jan. 15, 2003.
57. Interview, Craig Miner with Dr. Clark Ahlberg, May 25, 1994.
58. Interview Craig Miner with Dr. Fred Sudermann, Mar. 12, 2003.
59. For background, see Craig Miner, *Studying to Care: A History of the Wesley Medical Research Institutes, 1949–1999* (Wichita: Wesley Medical Research Institutes, 2000); Dr. Howard Clark and Craig Miner, *A History of the Medical Society of Sedgwick County* 2 vols. (Wichita: Medical Society of Sedgwick County, 2001, 2003); Hal Rothman, *A Tradition of Caring*, 1889–1989 (Wichita: St. Francis Regional Medical Center, 1988).
60. "Reflections, Charles E. Brackett, Jr., M.D.," 27.
61. Interview, Craig Miner with Dr. Joseph Meek, Feb. 19, 2003.
62. Interview, Craig Miner with Dr. Clark Ahlberg, May 25, 1994.
63. "Wichita State University: A University in Transition," December 1976, box 2a, Clark Ahlberg Papers, WSU archives, Special Collections, Wichita State University.
64. Craig Miner, interview with Dr. Charles Brackett, Feb. 1, 2004.
65. "Reflections. Charles E. Brackett, Jr., M.D.," 26–28.
66. Handwritten notes by Dr. Cramer Reed marked "for historical purposes," n.d. (c. 1970), Cramer Reed personal papers.
67. Dr. Cramer Reed to Dr. Charles Brackett, May 18, 1970, file 1B1, KUSM-W archives.
68. Dr. Jack Walker to Dr. Cramer Reed, July 30, 1970; Dr. Jack Walker to Dr. Homer Holt, Aug. 3, 1970, file IC8a, ibid.
69. Dr. Cramer Reed to Dr. Jack Walker, Oct. 1, 1970, ibid.
70. Dr. J.H. Holt to Dr. Cramer Reed, Sept. 16, 1970, ibid.
71. Dr. Lew Purinton to Dr. Cramer Reed, Jan. 7, 1971, ibid.
72. Interview, Craig Miner with Dr. Lew Purinton, Mar. 24, 2003.
73. Dr. Cramer Reed to Dr. Lester Garfinkel, Sept. 11, 1970, file 8A, KUSM-W archives.

74. Dr. Daniel Roberts to Dr. Kermit Krantz, Sept. 30, 1971, ibid.
75. *Fredonia Daily Herald*, Nov. 19, 1970, clippings file, KUSM-W archives.
76. *Manhattan Mercury*, Nov. 19, 1970, ibid.
77. *Kansas City Kansan*, Nov. 19, 1970, ibid.
78. *Wichita Eagle*, Nov. 19, 1970, ibid.
79. *Sunflower* (Wichita State University), Nov. 20, 1970, ibid.
80. *MSSC News* (Feb., 1971). *Wichita Beacon*, Mar. 5, 1971, clippings file, KUSM-W archives.
81. *Wichita Beacon*, Mar. 5, 1971, clippings file, KUSM-W archives.
82. *Wichita Eagle*, June 1, 1971, ibid.
83. *Wichita Beacon*, Mar. 5, 1971, ibid.
84. *Iola Register*, May 17, 1971, ibid.
85. *Wichita Beacon*, June 28, 1971, ibid.
86. Interview, Craig Miner with Dr. William Rieke, Mar. 5, 2003.
87. "Reflections. William O. Rieke, M.D." in Friesen and Hudson, *The Kansas School of Medicine*, 30–31.
88. Dr. Cramer Reed to Dr. Jack Walker, Feb. 9, 1971, file IC8a, KUSM-W archives.
89. Reed notes, June 11, 1971, ibid.
90. Interview, Craig Miner with Dr. E. Lawrence Chalmers, July 14, 2003.
91. Meeting notes, July 13, 1971, file IC8a, KUSM-W archives.
92. "Draft for Discussion with Wichita Groups," signed Russell Mills, Ph.D., Associate Dean and William Rieke, M.D. Vice Chancellor and the KUMC ad hoc Committee for Affiliations, file 1B1, ibid.
93. Interview, Craig Miner with Dr. William Rieke, Mar. 5, 2003.
94. Notes on legislative action 1971–72, Cramer Reed personal papers.
95. "Medical School Feasibility Study: An Approach for Consideration," file 1A2B, KUSM-W archives.
96. Dr. William Reals to Dr. Oliver Ebel, Aug. 3, 1971, ibid.
97. Richard Egan to Dr. William Reals, Sept. 9, 1971. James Cavenaugh to Dr. James Donnell, Sept. 20, 1971, ibid.
98. Meeting notes, Sept. 2, 1971, Cramer Reed personal papers.
99. *Iola Register*, Sept. 18, 1971, clippings file, KUSM-W archives.
100. *Kansas City Kansan*, Sept. 22, 1971, ibid.

—Chapter Three—

101. Interview, Craig Miner with Dwight Allen, Jan. 14, 2003.
102. Interview, Craig Miner with Dr. Phillip Burnstorf [sp], Mar. 19, 2003.
103. Interview, Craig Miner with Dr. Ernest Crow, Jan. 14, 2003.
104. Interview, Craig Miner with Maysel White, Jan. 15, 2003.
105. Interview, Craig Miner with Dr. Dean Kortge, Jan. 22, 2003.
106. Interview, Craig Miner with Dr. Garold Minns, Apr. 29, 2003.
107. Interview, Craig Miner with Dr. George Farha, Jan. 21, 2003.
108. Interview, Craig Miner with Marlin Rein, Jan. 29, 2003.
109. Interview, Craig Miner with Dr. Fred Sudermann, Mar. 12, 2003.
110. Interview, Craig Miner with Dr. Loren Welch, Feb. 12, 2003.
111. Interview, Craig Miner with Hazel Fenske, Jan. 15, 2003.
112. *Wichita Beacon*, Sept. 23, 1971, clippings file, KUSM-W archives.
113. *Wichita Beacon*, Sept. 24, 1971, ibid.
114. *Salina Journal*, Sept. 24, Oct. 5, 1971, ibid. Charles Pearson in *Wichita Eagle and*

Beacon Magazine, Oct. 3, 1971, ibid.

115. *Lawrence Daily Journal-World*, Sept. 25, 1971, ibid.
116. *Russell Record*, Sept. 27, 1971, ibid.
117. *Emporia Gazette*, Sept. 27, 1971, ibid.
118. Docking quoted in *Pratt Tribune*, Jan. 14, 1972, ibid.
119. Charles Pearson in *Wichita Eagle and Beacon Magazine*, Oct. 3, 1971, ibid. Reuben Burkan letter in *Chanute Tribune*, Oct. 5, 1971, ibid.
120. *Emporia Times*, Oct. 6, 1971, ibid.
121. *Medical Center Bulletin* (Oct., 1971), ibid.
122. *Wichita Eagle*, Oct. 10, 1971, ibid.
123. *Wichita Eagle*, Dec. 17, 1971, ibid.
124. *Arkansas City Traveler*, Nov. 5, 1971, ibid.
125. W.O. Rieke to Applicants for 1972 Freshman Medical Class, Dec. 27, 1971, file 1C3e, KUSM-W archives.
126. Interview, Craig Miner with Dr. Archie Dykes, Apr. 2, 2003.
127. Interview, Craig Miner with Dr. William Rieke, Mar. 5, 2003. Interview, Craig Miner with Patricia Head, May 12, 2003.
128. *Cunningham Clipper*, Mar. 30, 1972, in clippings file, KUSM-W archives.
129. *Wichita Eagle and Beacon*, Feb. 14, 1972, ibid.
130. *Kansas City Times*, Feb. 26, 1972, ibid. An excellent overview of the development of the "newer" facility and the rather parallel struggle with the state legislature in the 1920s to improve the facilities is Sims, *The Wahl Years.*
131. Cramer Reed to Russell Nelson, Feb. 17, 1972, file 8A, KUSM-W archives.
132. *Lawrence Journal*, Feb. 19, 1972, in clippings files, KUSM-W archives.
133. *Russell Daily News*, Feb. 1, 1972, ibid.
134. Interview, Craig Miner with Dr. Lew Purinton, Mar. 24, 2003.
135. W.F. McGuire in *Wichita Eagle*, Feb. 3, 1972, in clippings file, KUSM-W archives.
136. Reed to McGuire, Feb. 18, 1972, file 1C8, ibid.
137. Wichita Chamber of Commerce to Ahlberg and Reed, Nov. 8, 1971, file 1C8A, KUSM-W archives.
138. Monte Johnson to Reed, Aug. 11, 1972, in clippings file, KUSM-W archives.
139. Larry Jones to Archie Dykes, May 31, 1978, file 1B2d, ibid.
140. See for example Cramer Reed to Clyde Reed, Feb. 21, 1972, file 1C8A, ibid.
141. Cramer Reed to Robert Evans, Oct. 3, 1973, file 1C8D, ibid.
142. Robert Evans to Cramer Reed, Oct. 9, 1972, ibid.
143. Interview, Craig Miner with Dr. Cramer Reed, Jan. 7, 2003.
144. Ibid.
145. Interview, Craig Miner with Dr. Archie Dykes, Apr. 2, 2003.
146. Interview, Craig Miner with Marlin Rein, Jan. 29, 2003.
147. Interview, Craig Miner with Dr. Archie Dykes, Apr. 2, 2003.
148. Interview, Craig Miner with Dr. John Breazeale, Feb. 5, 2003.
149. William Rieke to Howard Feldman, Apr. 23, 1972, file 1C3B, KUSM-W archives.
150. Reed to R.W. Roskens, Dec. 29, 1971, file 1C8E, ibid. Simon Pollack to Reed, Jan. 24, 1972, file 1C8A, ibid. Steven Beering to Reed, May 9, 1972, file 1C8E, ibid. Richard Moy to Reed, June 12, 1972, file 1C8A, ibid. Wendell Smith to Reed, Nov. 27, 1972, ibid. Robert Evans to Reed, Oct. 9, 1973, file 1C8D, ibid.
151. Dr. Ernest Crow confirms this. Interview, Craig Miner with Dr. Ernest Crow, Jan. 14, 2003.
152. William Mallon, Mandy Lieu, Robert Jones, Michael Whitcomb, *Mini-Med: The Role of Regional Campuses in U.S. Medical Education* (Washington, D.C.: Association for American Medical Colleges, 2003), 1, 6, 10, 23, 33, 35.

153. Prime examples are Dr. Gayle Stephens, of the Department of Family Practice at the Wichita institution, who moved to the Huntsville campus of the University of Alabama School of Medicine (authorized 1971) and Dr. Robert Manning, who was first with KUMC, then the KUSM-W and later at a similar model medical school in Norfolk, VA. Interview, Craig Miner with Dr. Gayle Stevens, Feb. 3, 2003; Interview Craig Miner with Dr. Robert Manning, Feb. 24, 2003.
154. "The Origins and Conceptual Development of the Southern Illinois School of Medicine," p. 4, enclosed in Richard Moy to Cramer Reed, June 12, 1972, file 1C8A, KUSM-W archives.
155. Reed, speech notes, July 18, 1972, ibid.
156. To avoid confusion, henceforth the school will be referred to generally as KUSM-W, while mentioning in appropriate places the evolution of the name changes.
157. William Rieke to Cramer Reed, Oct. 5, 1972, file 1A3, KUSM-W archives.
158. McDill Boyd to William Rieke, Nov. 13, 1972, file 1C3C, ibid. William Rieke to Wes Sowers, copies to other politicians, Jan. 19, 1973, file 1C3A, ibid.
159. Cramer Reed to Clyde Reed, Feb. 21, 1973, file 1C3A, ibid.
160. Cramer Reed to Clyde Reed, Feb. 28, 1973, ibid.
161. *Wichita Eagle*, May 18, 1972, clippings file, KUSM-W archives.
162. *Wichita Eagle*, July 22, 1972, ibid.

—Chapter Four—

163. *Wichita Eagle*, Aug. 20, 1972, clippings file, KUSM-W archives. Crow, "Department of Internal Medicine," 2.
164. Interview, Craig Miner with Roy House, May 5, 2003.
165. Interview, Craig Miner with Dr. George Platt, Mar. 12, 2003.
166. *Wichita Eagle*, n.d. [Oct., 1972], clippings file, KUSM-W archives.
167. *Wichita Eagle*, Nov. 17, 1972, ibid.
168. *Wichita Eagle*, Sept. 28, 1972, ibid.
169. Ibid., Nov. 4, 1972.
170. Ibid., Mar. 23, 1973.
171. Ibid., Nov. 27, 1972.
172. Ibid., n.d. [early 1973].
173. *Wichita Beacon*, Feb. 16, 1973, ibid.
174. *Wichita Eagle*, Feb. 14, 1973, ibid.
175. Ibid., Mar. 21, 1973.
176. Ibid., Nov. 16, 1973.
177. *MSSC News*, June 1, 1973, ibid. *Wichita Eagle*, Sept. 9, 1973, ibid.
178. *Wichita Eagle*, Feb. 18, 1973, ibid.
179. Interview, Craig Miner with Hazel Fenske, Jan. 15, 2003.
180. Interview, Craig Miner with Dr. Richard Guthrie, Feb. 3, 2003.
181. Interview, Craig Miner with Jerry Lessard, Jan. 21, 2003.
182. Interview, Craig Miner with RoxAnn Dicker, May 25, 2003.
183. *Lawrence Daily Journal*, Aug. 24, 1973, clippings file, KUSM-W archives.
184. *Fredonia Daily Herald*, Sept. 26, 1973, ibid.
185. Interview, Craig Miner with Dr. Robert Manning, Feb. 24, 2003.
186. Interview, Craig Miner with Dr. Joseph Meek, Feb. 19, 2003.
187. Interview, Craig Miner with Dr. Gayle Stephens, Feb. 3, 2003.
188. Kellerman, et al., *In Their Own Words*, xiv.
189. Cramer Reed to Gayle Stephens, July 3, 1972, file 8A, KUSM-W archives.

190. Cramer Reed to Daniel Roberts, July 10, 1972, ibid.
191. Cramer Reed to members of MSSC, Oct. 6, 1972, ibid.
192. Cramer Reed to George Farha, Sept. 7, 1973, ibid. List of clinical associates, Feb. 8, 1974, ibid.
193. Cramer Reed to Russell Nelson, Jan. 22, 1974, ibid.
194. Interview, Craig Miner with Dr. Richard Guthrie, Feb. 3, 2003. For more on Guthrie and the general history of pediatric medicine in Wichita, see Craig Miner, *Mirrors of Heaven: Babies, Children & Pediatric Medicine in Wichita, 1870–2000* (Wichita: Wesley Medical Research Institutes, 2001).
195. Interview, Craig Miner with Dr. Ernest Crow, Jan. 14, 2003. Crow, "Department of Internal Medicine," 3–4. Interview, Craig Miner with Dr. Richard Guthrie, Feb. 3, 2003.
196. *Lawrence Journal World*, Feb. 14, 1973, clippings file, KUSM-W archives.
197. Interview, Craig Miner with Dr. George Farha, Jan. 21, 2003. For more on Roberts's background, see Miner, *Studying to Care*, 63–78.
198. Interview, Craig Miner with Dr. Robert Manning, Feb. 24, 2003.
199. Interview, Craig Miner with Roy House, May 5, 2003. Interview, Craig Miner with Dr. Robert Manning, Feb. 24, 2003.
200. "Daniel K. Roberts, M.D." Store Box 1, University Relations, KUSM-W archives.
201. *Wichita Eagle*, Apr. 19, 1981, clippings file, KUSM-W archives.
202. Interview, Craig Miner with Maggie Roberts, Jan. 8, 2003.
203. Interview, Craig Miner with Dr. Dean Schwartz, Feb. 24, 2003.
204. William Rieke to Wes Sowards and others, Jan. 19, 1973, file 1C3C, KUSM-W archives.
205. Interview, Craig Miner with Dr. George Dyck, Mar. 14, 2003.
206. *MSSC News*, June 1, 1973, clippings file, KUSM-W archives.
207. Interview, Craig Miner with Vince Marshall, Jan. 7, 2003.
208. Interview, Craig Miner with Jerry Lessard, Jan. 21, 2003.
209. Interview, Craig Miner with RoxAnn Dicker, June 25, 2003.
210. Interview, Craig Miner with Dean Kortge, Jan. 22, 2003.
211. Interview, Craig Miner with Dr. Joseph Dominic, July 17, 2003.
212. Interview, Craig Miner with Lorene Valentine, July 30, 2003.
213. *WSU News*, Apr. 28, 1972, KUSM-W archives.
214. Ibid., May 5, 1972.
215. Ibid., Oct. 20, 1972.
216. Ibid., Nov. 3, 1972.
217. Ibid., Sept. 29, 1972.
218. Ibid., Nov. 3, 1972.
219. Ibid. Feb. 2, Feb. 16, 1973.
220. Draft for article, June 12, 1973, file 1C8E, KUSM-W archives.
221. Cramer Reed to William Rieke, Aug. 10, 1973, file 1C3C, ibid.
222. *Wichita Eagle*, n.d. [early 1973], clippings file, ibid.
223. Cramer Reed to Robert Evans, Oct. 3, 1973, file 1C8D, ibid.
224. Robert Evans to Cramer Reed, Oct. 9, 1973, ibid.
225. [*Sunflower*], n.d. [early 1973], clippings file, vol. 1, ibid.
226. *MSSC News* (July 1973), clippings file, ibid.
227. *Wichita Eagle*, Sept. 9, 1973, ibid.
228. *Andover Journal*, Jan. 3, 1974, ibid.
229. *Lawrence Journal World*, Jan. 26, 1974, ibid.
230. *Phillipsburg Review*, Feb. 21, 1974, ibid.
231. *Wichita Eagle*, Feb. 12, 1974, ibid.
232. Ibid., Feb. 15, 1974.
233. Cramer Reed to William Brown, Sept. 12, 1974, KUSM-W archives.

234. Interview, Craig Miner with Dr. Kent Murray, June 30, 2003.
235. Interview, Craig Miner with Dr. Garold Minns, Apr. 29, 2003. For background on KU at this time, see Rusty Monhollon, *'This is America?': The Sixties in Lawrence, Kansas* (New York: Palgrave, 2002).
236. Interview, Craig Miner with Dr. Robert Manning, Feb. 24, 2003.
237. Interview, Craig Miner with Dr. R. Lawrence Sifford, June 18, 2003.
238. An example was neurologist Dr. Lauren Welch. Interview, Craig Miner with Dr. Lauren Welch, Feb. 12, 2003.
239. These insights come from: Interview, Craig Miner with Dr. Sheldon Preskorn, May 14, 2003.
240. *Sunflower*, Sept. 30, 1974, ibid.

—Chapter Five—

241. "New Beginnings: The Wichita State University Branch, Kansas University School of Medicine," n.d. [June 1974], file 1A3, KUSM-W archives.
242. Wesley Sowers to Dr. Archie Dykes, Apr. 17, 1974, file 1B2A, ibid.
243. Dr. Cramer Reed to Dr. Robert Evans, Oct. 21, 1974, file 1C8D, ibid.
244. *Wichita Eagle*, Mar. 17, 1975, clippings file, ibid.
245. Goals Fiscal Year 1975, file 1C3D, ibid.
246. Dr. William Rieke to Dr. Cramer Reed, Nov. 12, 1974, ibid.
247. Dr. William Rieke to Dr. Cramer Reed, Nov. 12, 1974, file 1C3D, ibid.
248. Dr. Cramer Reed to Dr. George Burkett, Apr. 14, 1975, file 1C8B, ibid.
249. Dr. Cramer Reed to Dr. Archie Dykes, Jan. 21, 1976, ibid.
250. *KU Faculty and Staff Newsletter*, Sept. 8, 1975, clippings file, ibid. A useful compilation of key dates in the earlier history of the school was compiled by Lorene Valentine, Sept. 18, 1981 and is found in the KUSM-W archives.
251. Dr. Cramer Reed to William Brown, Sept. 12, 1974, file 1C8B, ibid.
252. Dr. Cramer Reed to Dr. David Robinson, July 16, 1975, file 1C4, ibid.
253. Dr. David Robinson to Dr. Clark Ahlberg, July 17, 1975, ibid.
254. J.D. to D.C.R., Feb. 20, 1976, file 1C5A, ibid.
255. *Lawrence Journal-World*, Nov. 21, 1975, clippings file, KUSM-W archives.
256. *Harper Advocate*, Jan. 23, 1975, ibid.
257. *Anthony Republican*, Feb. 26, 1975, ibid.
258. *Wichita Eagle*, June 10, 1975, ibid.
259. *Sunflower*, Mar. 10, 1976, ibid.
260. *Howard Courant-Citizen*, Jan. 23, 1975, ibid.
261. *Wichita Eagle*, Mar. 17, 1975, ibid.
262. Ibid., Mar. 18, 1975.
263. *The Branch Log*, May 12, 1976, KUSM-W archives.
264. *Wichita Eagle*, July 11, 1975, clippings file, KUSM-W archives.
265. *Junction City Daily Union*, Sept. 30, 1975, ibid.
266. *The Branch Log*, Sept. 10, 1975, KUSM-W archives.
267. Ibid., Feb. 12, 1976.
268. Ibid., Oct. 10, 1975.
269. Ibid., Sept. 10, 1975, Jan. 9, 1976.
270. Ibid., Nov. 12, 1975.
271. Ibid., Jan. 9, 1976.
272. Ibid., Jan. 9, 1976.
273. Ibid., Jan. 9, Feb. 12, Mar. 12, May 12, 1976.

274. *Belle Plaine News*, Oct. 22, 1975, clippings file, ibid. Kinsley Mercury, Sept. 23, 1976, ibid.
275. *The Jayhawk Family Physician* (July 1976), ibid.
276. *Cunningham Clipper*, Oct. 21, 1976, ibid.
277. *Wichita Eagle*, Oct. 2, 1977; Parsons Sun, Nov. 16, 1977, ibid.
278. Interview, Craig Miner with Dr. Dean Kortge, Jan. 22, 2003.
279. Interview, Craig Miner with Dr. Archie Dykes, Apr. 2, 2003.
280. Interview, Craig Miner with Dr. David Waxman, Apr. 14, 2003. "Reflections. David Waxman, M.D." in Friesen and Hudson, *The Kansas School of Medicine*, 34–35.
281. The phrase comes from: Interview, Craig Miner with Dr. Anne Walling, May 12, 2003.
282. Dr. Archie Dykes to Dr. Cramer Reed, Aug. 30, 1975, file 1B2A, KUSM-W archives.
283. Memo, July 1975, Reed personal papers.
284. Dr. Clark Ahlberg to Dr. Archie Dykes, Sept. 9, 1975, ibid.
285. Dr. Archie Dyke to Dr. Clark Ahlberg, Sept. 14, 1975, ibid.
286. Notes for meeting with C.A. [Clark Ahlberg], Dec. 1975, ibid.
287. Interview, Craig Miner with Dr. Cramer Reed, Jan. 7, 2003.
288. Interview, Craig Miner with Dr. George Dyke, Mar. 14, 2003.
289. Interview, Craig Miner with Dr. Cramer Reed, Jan. 7, 2003. Dr. Guthrie gave me some insights into the private practice problems. Interview, Craig Miner with Dr. Richard Guthrie, Feb. 3, 2003.
290. Dr. Cramer Reed to Archie Dykes, Mar. 5, 1976, file 1B2B, KUSM-W archives.
291. Dr. Cramer Reed to Dr. Donald Albers, Apr. 1, 1976, "chronological" notebooks, ibid.
292. Dr. Cramer Reed to Dr. Daniel Carr, Apr. 27, 1976, ibid.

—Chapter Six—

293. Kugel speech, May 12, 1976, file 1C5A, KUSM-W archives.
294. Dr. Cramer Reed to Dr. Richard Walsh, June 1, 1976, "chronological notebooks," KUSM-W archives.
295. Interview, Craig Miner with Dr. Richard Walsh, June 4, 2003.
296. *Wichita Eagle*, Mar. 2, 1977, clippings file, KUSM-W archives. Dr. Cramer Reed to Dr. Ernest Crow, July 30, 1976, "chronological notebooks," KUSM-W archives.
297. Dr. Cramer Reed to Dr. Archie Dykes, Aug. 3, 1976, ibid.
298. Interview, Craig Miner with Dr. Richard Walsh, June 4, 2003.
299. Speech at Alpha Epsilon Delta initiation, May 8, 1976, file 1C8E, KUSM-W archives.
300. Dr. Robert Hudson, speech at Faculty Convocation, University of Kansas, Dec. 4, 1980, file 1A3, ibid.
301. Dr. Cramer Reed to Dr. John Breazeale, Mar. 10, 1975, Reed personal papers.
302. Dr. Cramer Reed to Dr. Clark Ahlberg, May 17, 1975, ibid.
303. Mission statement, July, 1975, ibid.
304. Dr. Archie Dykes to Dr. Cramer Reed, Jan. 3, 1975, Records of Chancellor's Office, Correspondence 1975, Series 2/15, box 8.
305. Dr. Archie Dykes to Dr. Tom Alderson, Apr. 6, 1975, ibid.
306. Dr. Archie Dykes to John Eberhardt, Apr. 6, 1975, ibid.
307. Dr. Archie Dykes to Don Boyett, Apr. 23, 1975, ibid.
308. Dr. Archie Dykes to Dr. Russell Mills, Sept. 28, 1975, ibid.
309. *Wichita Eagle*, July 19, 1976, clippings file, KUSM-W archives.
310. *Neodesha Daily Sun*, Mar. 24, 1976, ibid.
311. Dr. Cramer Reed to Dr. Clark Ahlberg, Dec. 14, 1976, Reed personal papers.
312. Dr. Cramer Reed to Hon. Theodore Cribbs, Nov. 1, 1976, "chronological note books," KUSM-W archives.

313. Minutes, Nov. 16, 1976, file 1C5A, KUSM-W archives.
314. Dr. Robert Kugel to Committee, Dec. 15, 1976, ibid.
315. Dr. Cramer Reed to Dr. Robert Kugel, Nov. 24, 1976, "chronological" notebooks, ibid.
316. Dr. Cramer Reed to Dr. Archie Dykes, Dec. 13, 1976, file 1B2B, ibid.
317. Dr. Cramer Reed to Dr. Archie Dykes, Dec. 27, 1976, "chronological" notebooks, ibid.
318. Dr. Cramer Reed to Dr. Clark Ahlberg, Jan. 13, 1977, Reed personal papers.
319. Larry Jones to Clark Ahlberg, June 23, 1977, ibid. This letter is also in the Ahlberg papers at WSU.
320. Dr. Cramer Reed to Dr. Archie Dykes, Dec. 13, 1976,"chonological" notebooks, KUSM-W archives.
321. Dr. Archie Dykes to Dr. Cramer Reed, Dec. 14, 1976, file 1B2C2, ibid.
322. Interview, Craig Miner with Dr. Anne Walling, May 12, 2003.
323. Interview, Craig Miner with RoxAnn Dicker, June 25, 2003.
324. Dr. Cramer Reed to Dr. Clark Ahlberg, July 19, 1977, "chronological" notebooks, KUSM-W archives.
325. *Wichita Eagle*, Mar. 31, 1978, clippings file, ibid.
326. Especially graphic and negative descriptions came from: Interviews, Craig Miner with Vince Marshall, Jan. 7, 2003; with Hazel Fenske, Jan. 15, 2003; with Barbara Delhotal, Jan. 8, 2003; with Maysel White, Jan. 15, 2003; with Dr. Richard Guthrie, Feb. 3, 2003.
327. Interview, Craig Miner with Jerry Lessard, Jan. 21, 2003.
328. *Wichita Beacon*, July 19, 1978, clippings file, KUSM-W archives.
329. Interview, Craig Miner with Maysel White, Jan. 15, 2003.
330. *Sunflower*, Nov. 8, 1976, clippings file, KUSM-W archives.
331. Dr. Cramer Reed to Dr. Clark Ahlberg, June 9, 1977, "chronological notebooks," ibid.
332. Timeline, "History of the University of Kansas School of Medicine-Wichita" by Lorene Valentine, Sept. 18, 1981.
333. Dr. Cramer Reed to Marlin Rein, June 28, 1977, "chronological notebooks," KUSM-W archives.
334. Dr. Archie Dykes to Hon. Mike Meacham, Aug. 22, 1977, file 1B2C2, ibid.
335. Interview, Craig Miner with Marlin Rein, Jan. 29, 2003.
336. Craig Miner, interview with Dr. George Platt, Mar. 12, 2003.
337. Press release, Aug. 29, 1977, file 1C7A2, KUSM-W archives.
338. Dr. Archie Dykes to faculty, staff, and students, Sept. 2, 1977, file 1B2C2, ibid.
339. Dr. Cramer Reed to Dr. Archie Dykes, Oct. 10, 1977, ibid.
340. Dr. Richard Walsh to Robert Van Citters, Apr. 12, 1978, file 1C7B1, ibid.
341. Dr. Archie Dykes to Dr. Cramer Reed, May 10, 1978, file 1B2D, ibid.
342. Dr. Cramer Reed to Dr. Joseph Meek, Jan. 9, 1977, file 1C8C1, ibid.
343. Dr. Cramer Reed to branch academic departments, Mar. 9, 1977, file 1B2C1, ibid.
344 Dr. Cramer Reed to Dr. Gayle Stephens, Mar. 17, 1977, "chronological" notebooks, ibid.
345. Dr. Cramer Reed to Dr. James Campbell, Mar. 29, 1977, ibid.
346. Dr. Archie Dykes to Dr. Cramer Reed, Apr. 9, 1977, file 1B2C1, ibid.
347. Dr. Cramer Reed to Dr. Archie Dykes, Apr. 22, 1977, "chronological" notebooks, ibid.
348. Dr. Cramer Reed to Dr. Clark Ahlberg, May 23, 1977, ibid.
349. Dr. Archie Dykes to Dr. Cramer Reed, June 22, 1977, file 1B2C1, ibid.
350. Dr. Cramer Reed to Dr. Archie Dykes, June ?, 1977, ibid.
351. Dr. Cramer Reed to Sister Bernadette, June 28, 1977, "chronological" notebooks, ibid.
352. Dr. Cramer Reed to Larry Jones, June 28, 1977, ibid.
353. Dr. Cramer Reed to Dwight Button, July 1, 1977, ibid.
354. Dr. Cramer Reed to Dr. Archie Dykes, July 14, 1977, file 1B2C2, ibid.
355. Dr. Cramer Reed to Terry Scanlon, July 19, 1977, "chronological" notebooks, ibid.

356. Dr. Cramer Reed to Dr. Archie Dykes, July 29, 1977, file 1B2C2, ibid.
357. Dr. Archie Dykes to Dr. Cramer Reed, Aug. 28, 1977, ibid.
358. Press release, Aug. 29, 1977, file 1C7A2, ibid.
359. Dr. Cramer Reed to Dr. Archie Dykes, Sept. 2, 1977, ibid.
360. Dr. Cramer Reed to Doris Geitgey, Oct. 7, 1977, file 1C8C1, ibid.
361. Dr. Cramer Reed to Dr. Archie Dykes, Oct. 10, 1977, file 1B2C2, ibid. See also Dr. Cramer Reed to Hon. Wesley Sowers, Oct. 18, 1977, file 1C8C1, ibid. on this issue.
362. Dr. Cramer Reed to Dr. Archie Dykes, Oct. 15, 1977, file 1B2C2, ibid.
363. Dr. Archie Dykes to Leonard Levand, Nov. 12, 1977, ibid.
364. Dr. Cramer Reed to department chairs, Dec. 19, 1977, "chronological" notebooks, ibid.
365. Dr. Richard Walsh to Dr. Robert Van Citters, Apr. 12, 1978, file 1C7B1, ibid.
366. Dr. Richard Walsh to Dr. David Waxman, Mar. 22, 1978, ibid. Dr. David Waxman to Dr. Richard Walsh, file 1C6B1, ibid.
367. Dr. Cramer Reed to Dr. Archie Dykes, Apr. 13, 1978, file 1B2D, ibid.
368. Dr. Richard Walsh to department chairs, May 18, 1978, file 1C7B1, ibid.
369. Dr. Cramer Reed to Dr. David Waxman, Mar. 31, 1978, file 1C6B1, ibid.
370. White Paper, Mar. 8, 1978, file 1C7B1, ibid.
371. Dr. Cramer Reed to Dr. David Waxman, Mar. 9, 1978, ibid.
372. Interview, Craig Miner with Martin Rein, Jan. 29, 2003.
373. Dr. Cramer Reed to Dr. Archie Dykes, Mar. 13, 1978, file 1B2D, ibid.
374. Dr. Cramer Reed to Dr. James Rhatigan, Apr. 20, 1978, file 1C8C2, ibid.
375. Dr. Richard Walsh to Dr. David Waxman, Mar. 2, 1978, file 1C6B1, ibid.
376. Dr. Cramer Reed to Dr. Archie Dykes, May 4, 1978, file 1B2D, ibid.
377. Dr. Archie Dykes to Dr. Cramer Reed, May 10, 1978, ibid.
378. This impression comes from various interviews, including the one with Reed himself, who said he "understands it better now than he did then." It is still, however, a sensitive issue, and interviewees did not talk about it in detail. There is nothing in the archives to suggest Reed was fired, but then one would not expect there would be.
379. Dr. Richard Walsh to Ann Bliss, May 12, 1978, file 1C7B1, ibid.
380. *The Monitor* (May/June 1978), ibid.
381. Interview, Craig Miner with Kent Murray, June 30, 2003.
382. Dr. Cramer Reed to Dr. Gayle Stephens, June 14, 1978, file 1C8C2, ibid.

—Chapter Seven—

383. Self Study 1978, LCME Study Task Force Committee, KUSM-W archives.
384. "University of Kansas School of Medicine-Wichita Faculty P.A. Professional Fee Income," file 8G1, ibid.
385. Dr. Douglas Voth to Dr. Cramer Reed, Mar. 6, 1978, ibid.
386. Interview, Craig Miner with Jerry Lessard, Jan. 21, 2003.
387. *Wichita Eagle*, May 5, 1978, clippings file, ibid.
388. Ibid., May 7, 1978.
389. Ibid., May 12, 1978.
390. *Topeka State Journal*, Sept. 19, 1978, ibid.
391. *Wichita Eagle*, Nov. 15, 1978, ibid. Ernest Crow to Richard Walsh, Jan. 10, 1979, file 1C7C1, KUSM archives.
392. *Wichita Eagle*, Oct. 13, 1978, clippings file, ibid.
393. *Wichita Beacon*, Nov. 15, 1978, ibid.
394. *Wichita Eagle*, May 12, 1978, ibid.
395. Dr. C.T. Hagen to Archie Dykes, May 10, 1978, file 1B2D, ibid.
396. Dr. Richard Walsh to Dr. David Waxman, May 31, 1978, file 1C7B1, ibid.

397. Dr. Douglas Voth to Richard Walsh, June 28, 1978, ibid.
398. Larry Jones to Dr. Archie Dykes, May 31, 1978, file 1B2D, ibid.
399. *Wichita Eagle*, July 13, 1978, clippings file, ibid.
400. Dr. Cramer Reed to Hon. Wesley Sowers, June 14, 1978, file 1C8C2, ibid.
401. Fred Weaver to Ed Kessinger of *Fredonia Daily Herald*, July 27, 1978, file 1B2D, ibid.
402. Dr. Richard Walsh, "The Medical School Present and Future," speech to Medical Society of Sedgwick County, December 5, 1978, file 1C7B2, ibid.
403. Interview, Craig Miner with Dr. Richard Walsh, June 4, 2003.
404. Dr. Richard Walsh to Herbert Pahl, Jan. 25, 1979, file 1C7C1, KUSM-W archives.
405. Dr. Richard Walsh to David Waxman, Apr. 17, 1979, ibid.
406. Walsh speech to Medical Education Association, June 21, 1979, ibid.
407. Dr. Richard Walsh to David Waxman, July 20, 1979, file 1C7C2, ibid.
408. *Monitor*, Nov./Dec., 1979, ibid.
409. Dr. Richard Walsh to David Waxman, Aug. 6, 1979, file 1C7C2, ibid.
410. Dr. Cramer Reed to Dr. Richard Walsh, June 1, 1979, file 1C8E, ibid.
411. Dr. Cramer Reed to Jordan Haines, Aug. 16, 1979, file 1C8C2, ibid.
412. Dr. Richard Walsh to David Waxman, Aug. 24, 1979, file 1C7C2, ibid.
413. Dr. Archie Dykes to Paul Wunsch, Sept. 12, 1979, file 1B2E, ibid.
414. Interview, Craig Miner with Dr. Anne Walling, Apr. 12, 2003.
415. Interview, Craig Miner with Barbara Delhotal, Jan. 8, 2003.
416. Interview, Craig Miner with Dr. David Street, Mar. 10, 2003.
417. Interview, Craig Miner with Vince Marshall, Jan. 7, 2003.
418. Interview, Craig Miner with Dr. Anne Walling, Apr. 12, 2003.
419. Interview, Craig Miner with Barbara Delhotal, Jan. 8, 2003. *Wichita Eagle*, July 28, 1981, clippings file, KUSM-W archives.
420. *Monitor*, Mar./Apr., 1979, KUSM-W archives.
421. Interview, Craig Miner with Dr. Dean Kortge, Jan. 22, 2003.
422. Interview, Craig Miner with Dr. Lauren Welch, Feb. 12, 2003.
423. Dr. Richard Walsh to Dr. David Waxman, May 5, 1980, file 1C7D, KUSM-W archives.
424. Interview, Craig Miner with Dr. Richard Walsh, June 4, 2003.
425. Dr. William Reals to William Wiese, Sept. 8, 1981, file 1C7D, ibid.
426. *Wichita Eagle*, Mar. 20, 1981, clippings file, KUSM-W archives.
427. Interview, Craig Miner with Dr. Gene Budig, Apr. 2, 2003.
428. Interview, Craig Miner with Dr. Anne Walling, May 12, 2003.
429. Interview, Craig Miner with RoxAnn Dicker, May 25, 2003.
430. Interview, Craig Miner with Jan Arbuckle, Mar. 10, 2003.
431. Interview, Craig Miner with Dr. Anne Walling, May 12, 2003.
432. Interview, Craig Miner with Lorene Valentine, July 30, 2003. *Wellington Daily News*, Apr. 10, 1981, clippings file, KUSM-W archives.
433. Interview, Craig Miner with Dr. Sechin Cho, May 7, 2003.
434. Interview, Craig Miner with Hazel Fenske, Jan. 15, 2003.
435. Interview, Craig Miner with Dr. Richard Shaw, Apr. 14, 2003.

—Chapter Eight—

436. Dr. Cramer Reed speech Nov. 6, 1980, file 1C8E, KUSM-W archives.
437. *Wichita Beacon*, May 3, 1979, clippings file, ibid.
438. Image Plan by James R. Reed, Oct. 15, 1981, file 1A3, KUSM-W archives.

439. Marilyn Cannday, "Playing the Odds," *The Wichitan* (August 1979): 75, clippings file, ibid.
440. *The Oread* (Aug. 1979), ibid.
441. *Goodland Daily Record*, Aug. 27, 1979, *Wellington Daily News*, Oct. 16, 1979, *Wichita Beacon*, Aug. 28, 1980, Ottawa Herald, Dec. 19, 1980, *Wichita Eagle*, Dec. 20, 1980, *University Daily Kansan*, Feb. 11, 1981, ibid. Interview, Craig Miner with Dr. Richard Guthrie, Feb. 3, 2003.
442. *Wichita Eagle*, Feb. 17, 1988, clippings file, KUSM-W archives.
443. Ibid., Feb. 21, 1988.
444. *Lawrence Journal-World*, July 2, 1989, ibid.
445. *Wichita Eagle*, Apr. 19, 1981, ibid.
446. Ibid., Apr. 7, 1988. Craig Miner, *Studying to Care: A History of Wesley Medical Research Institutes, 1949–1999* (Wichita, KS: Wesley Medical Research Institutes, 2000), 89–90.
447. *Wichita Business Journal*, July 7, 1986, clippings file, KUSM-W archives.
448. Ibid., June 13, 1988.
449. *Wichita Eagle*, Nov. 21, 1988, ibid.
450. Ibid., Aug 31, Sept. 3, 1990.
451. Ibid., Jan. 24, 1985.
452. Materials in letter Donald Stewart to Craig Miner, Feb. 4, 2004. An excellent summary is Kansas Health Foundation, *A Decade of Kansas Philanthropy: 1985–1995* published by the Foundation. Interview, Craig Miner with Donald Stewart, Feb. 3, 2003.
453. *Wichita Eagle*, Aug. 9, 1987, clippings file, KUSM-W archives.
454. Ibid., Aug. 17, 1987.
455. Clipping, no paper listed, Aug. 17, 1987, ibid.
456. Clipping, no paper listed [*Wichita Business Journal?*], Aug. 24, 1987, ibid.
457. *Wichita Eagle*, Oct. 8, 1987, ibid.
458. Miner, *Studying to Care*, 103.
459. *Wichita Eagle*, Aug. 6, 1990, clippings file, KUSM-W archives.
460. Ibid., Aug. 23, 1981.
461. *Wichita Beacon*, Oct. 8, 1979, ibid.
462. *Wichita Eagle*, Dec. 13, 1982, ibid.
463. *Herington Times*, July 12, 1984, ibid.
464. Interview, Craig Miner with Dr. Neil Roach, Feb. 29, 2003.
465. *Wichita Eagle*, July 14, 1984, clippings file, KUSM-W archives.
466. *University Daily Kansan*, Aug. 30, 1982, ibid.
467. *Wichita Eagle*, Sept. 23, 28, 1988, ibid.
468. Ibid., Sept. 26, 1988.
469. *Arkansas City Traveler*, Sept. 9, 1985; *Derby Daily Reporter*, Feb. 21, 1986; non identified clip, Sept. 13, 1985, *Wichita Eagle*, July 11, Dec. 6. 1988, ibid.
470. *Leoti Standard*, Aug. 21, 1980, ibid.
471. *Manhattan Mercury*, Nov. 6, 1987, ibid.
472. *Kinsley Mercury*, Apr. 9, 1981, ibid.
473. *Wichita Eagle*, Dec. 13, 1982, ibid.
474. *Plainville Times*, Mar. 7, 1985, ibid.
475. *Goodland Sherman County Herald*, Mar. 13, 1980, ibid.
476. *Salina Journal*, June 1, 1980, ibid.
477. *WaKeeney Western Kansas World*, Feb. 7, 1985, ibid.
478. *Russell Daily News*, Feb. 21, 1985, ibid.
479. Ibid. Apr. 16, 1985.
480. *Kinsley Mercury*, Apr. 16, 1981.

481. *Jetmore Republican*, Nov. 19, 1981.
482. *Liberal Southwest Daily Times*, Apr. 21, 1982.
483. *Wichita Eagle*, Apr. 30, 1986.
484. Nancy S. Nowlin, M.D. and Douglas W. Voth, M.D., "Basic Clerkship: Students in Internal Medicine on a Community Clinical Campus," *Journal, Kansas Medical Society* 80 (July 1979): 409–23.
485. *Wichita Eagle*, Sept. 17, 1988, clippings file, KUSM-W archives.
486. *Lawrence Journal-World*, Aug. 19, 1989, ibid.
487. *University Daily Kansan*, Apr. 3, 1989, ibid.
488. *Wichita Eagle*, Aug. 29, 1987, ibid.
489. *Wichita Business Journal*, Aug. 22, 1988, ibid.
490. *Wichita Eagle*, Aug. 21, 1988, ibid.
491. *Wichita Eagle*, Apr. 7, 1985, ibid. "The University of Kansas School of Medicine-Wichita: A Ten-Year Review of a Community-Based Medical School," file 1A3, KUSM-W archives.
492. *Wichita Eagle*, May 10, 1986, clippings file, KUSM-W archives.
493. "Daniel K. Roberts M.D.," storage box 1, University Relations, ibid.
494. *Lawrence Journal World*, Aug. 19, 1989, clippings file, ibid.
495. *Hiawatha Daily World*, July 6, 1990, *Wichita Business Journal*, Sept. 10, 1990, ibid.

—Chapter Nine—

496. Interview, Craig Miner with Dr. Joseph Meek, Feb. 19, 2003.
497. Interview, Craig Miner with Dr. Frederick Chang, May 22, 2003.
498. *Wichita Business Journal*, Nov. 12, 1990, clippings file, KUSM-W archives.
499. *Monitor*, Jan. 1991, KUSM-W archives.
500. Ibid.
501. Ibid., Mar. 1991.
502. Ibid., July 1992.
503. Ibid., Feb. 1994.
504. Ibid., June/July 2003.
505. Ibid., Jan. 1993.
506. Ibid., Jan. 1994.
507. Interview, Craig Miner with Barbara Delhotal, Jan. 8, 2003.
508. Interview, Craig Miner with Dr. Frederick Chang, May 22, 2003.
509. Interview, Craig Miner with Dr. Hewitt Goodpasture, Mar. 3, 2003.
510. Interview, Craig Miner with Dr. Richard Shaw, Apr. 14, 2003.
511. *Wichita Business Journal*, Nov. 12, 1990, clippings file, KUSM-W archives.
512. Interview, Craig Miner with Dr. Gene Budig, Apr. 2, 2003.
513. *Lawrence Journal World*, n.d. (Aug, 1991), clippings file, KUSM-W archives.
514. Interview, Craig Miner with RoxAnn Dicker, May 25, 2003.
515. Interview, Craig Miner with Dr. George Dyke, Mar. 14, 2003. Interview, Craig Miner with Dr. Sheldon Preskorn, May 14, 2003.
516. Interview, Craig Miner with Dr. Craig Molgaard, May 21, 2003.
517. Interview, Craig Miner with Dr. Sheldon Preskorn, May 14, 2003.
518. Interview, Craig Miner with Dr. Alex Ammar, May 21, 2003.
519. Interview, Craig Miner with Jan Arbuckle, Mar. 10, 2003.
520. *Wichita Business Journal*, Mar. 27, 1992, ibid.
521. Interview, Craig Miner with Dr. Garold Minns, Apr. 29, 2003. *Lawrence Journal World*, May 2, 1990, clippings file, KUSM-W archives.

522. Interview, Craig Miner with Dr. Lauren Welch, Feb. 12, 2003.
523. *Wichita Business Journal*, Nov. 12, 1990, clippings file, KUSM-W archives.
524. *Lawrence Journal World*, n.d. (Aug. 1991), ibid. Monitor, Nov. 1990, KUSM-W archives.
525. *Wichita Eagle*, Sept. 30, Oct. 3, 1992, clippings file, ibid.
526. *Kansas Connections*, Winter, 1994, KUSM-W archives.
527. Ibid., Autumn 1993.
528. Ibid.
529. Ibid.
530. Ibid.
531. Ibid.
532. *Emporia Gazette*, Nov. 20, 1992, clippings file, KUSM-W archives.
533. *Lawrence Journal World*, July 6, 1993, ibid.
534. *Wichita Eagle*, Feb. 7, 1993, ibid.
535. *Topics*, Jan. 5, 1994, ibid.
536. *Wichita Business Journal*, Jan. 28, 1994.
537. Ibid., Apr. 15, 1994.
538. *Wichita Eagle*, Sept. 29, Oct. 3, 1991, ibid.
539. Ibid., Dec. 21, 1995.
540. *Wichita Business Journal*, June 5, 1992, ibid.
541. Interview, Craig Miner with Sister Sylvia Egan, Mar. 24, 2003.
542. Interview, Craig Miner with Dr. Alex Ammar, May 21, 2003.
543. *Kansas Connections*, Autumn 1993, KUSM-W archives.
544. *Wichita Business Journal*, Aug. 6, 1993, clippings file, KUSM-W archives.
545. *Kansas Connections*, Autumn 1993.
546. *Wichita Eagle*, Nov. 15, 1993, clippings file, KUSM-W archives.
547. Interview, Craig Miner with Dr. Craig Molgaard, May 21, 2003.
548. Interview, Craig Miner with Dr. Edwards Dismuke, June 30, 2003.
549. The departmental information comes from the Annual Reports of the Department of Family and Community Medicine, KUSM-W archives.
550. *Independence News*, June 6, 1992, clippings file, ibid.
551. Interview, Craig Miner with Dr. Craig Molgaard, May 21, 2003.
552. Interview, Craig Miner with Dr. Edwards Dismuke, June 30, 2003.

—Chapter Ten—

553. *Wichita Eagle*, Mar. 18, 1995, Jan. 14, 1996, *Times-Sentinel* (Cheney), Apr. 25, 1996, clippings file, KUSM-W archives.
554. *Kansas Connections*, KUSM-W archives.
555. *Wichita Eagle*, June 8, 1995, clippings file, KUSM-W archives.
556. Ibid., Mar. 9, 1995.
557. Ibid., Mar. 2, 1997.
558. *Wichita Business Journal*, May 26, 1995, ibid.
559. Ibid., Apr. 26, 1996.
560. Ibid., July 5, 1996.
561. *Kansas Connections*, Autumn 1994, KUSM-W archives.
562. Ibid. Spring 1995.
563. *Monitor*, July 1996, ibid.
564. Ibid., May 1996.
565. *Wichita Business Journal*, Apr. 20, 1995, clippings file, KUSM-W archives.

566. *Wellington Daily News*, May 16, 1995, ibid.
567. For the history of the Kansas Health Foundation's origin and change, see Craig Miner, *Studying to Care*, 92–109.
568. *Wichita Eagle*, May 18, 1995, ibid.
569. *Monitor*, Apr., 1999, KUSM-W archives.
570. Ibid., Nov./Dec. 2000.
571. Ibid., Dec. 2001.
572. Ibid., June/July 2002.
573. Ibid., June/July 2003
574. *Times-Sentinel* (Cheney) Apr. 25, 1996, clippings file, KUSM-W archives.
575. *Hutchinson News*, n.d. (Mar., 1999), ibid.
576. Department of Family and Community Medicine, Annual Report, 1996, KUSM-W archives.
577. *Wichita Eagle*, Oct. 1, 1996, clippings file, KUSM-W archives.
578. Ibid., June 20, 2000.
579. *Monitor*, June 2001, KUSM-W archives.
580. *Kansas Connections*, Spring, 2001, ibid.
581. Ibid., Summer 2001.
582. *Monitor*, Jan. 2003, ibid.
583. Ibid., Aug. 2003.
584. KUSM-W, *Annual Report*, 2003, KUSM-W archives.
585. *Wichita Eagle*, June 8, 1995, clippings file, KUSM-W archives.

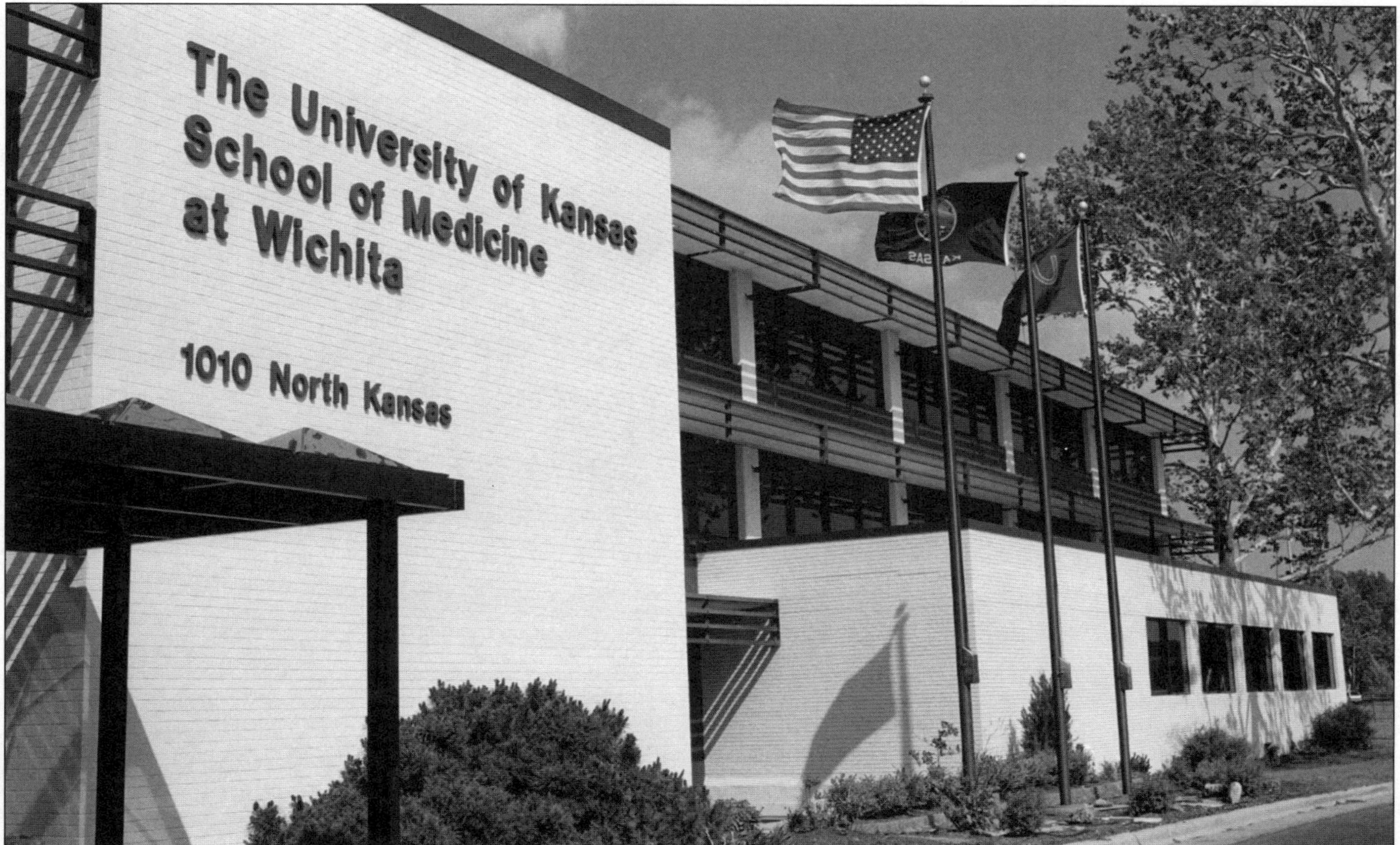

The University of Kansas School of Medicine - Wichita.

100 YEARS

1905·2005

KU School of Medicine

The University of Kansas School of Medicine
celebrated its 100th anniversary in 2005.

30 YEARS

1975-2005

KU SCHOOL OF MEDICINE WICHITA

The University of Kansas School of Medicine - Wichita celebrated its 30th anniversary in 2005.